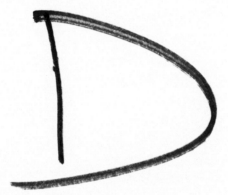

Walker Finds a Way

by the same author

Running with Walker
A Memoir
Robert Hughes
ISBN 978 1 84310 755 2
eISBN 978 1 84642 406 9

Walker Finds a Way

Running Into the Adult World with Autism

ROBERT HUGHES

Jessica Kingsley *Publishers*
London and Philadelphia

First published in 2016
by Jessica Kingsley Publishers
73 Collier Street
London N1 9BE, UK
and
400 Market Street, Suite 400
Philadelphia, PA 19106, USA

www.jkp.com

Library of Congress Cataloging in Publication Data
A CIP catalog record for this book is available from the Library of Congress

British Library Cataloguing in Publication Data
A CIP catalogue record for this book is available from the British Library

ISBN 978 1 78592 010 3
eISBN 978 1 78450 253 9

Printed and bound in the United States

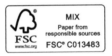

MIX
Paper from
responsible sources
FSC
www.fsc.org   FSC® C013483

FOR MY MOTHER, RUTH HUGHES ATKINS

Contents

CHAPTER 1 Zoo–Train–Walk: December 2013   9

CHAPTER 2 "What's Your Plan?": Winter 2007   25

CHAPTER 3 A Brave New World   41

CHAPTER 4 The Empty Nesters   55

CHAPTER 5 Friends   69

CHAPTER 6 "I Work There"   83

CHAPTER 7 Fence Me In   99

CHAPTER 8 A Very Un-Merry Birthday   113

CHAPTER 9 "People Change"   129

CHAPTER 10 Agitation: Father and Son   147

CHAPTER 11 Psycho Dad Makes a Personal Appearance   161

CHAPTER 12 Our Winter of Discontent   181

CHAPTER 13 Hold On, Partner   199

CHAPTER 14 The Escape Artist   217

CHAPTER 15 Afterword: July 2015   233

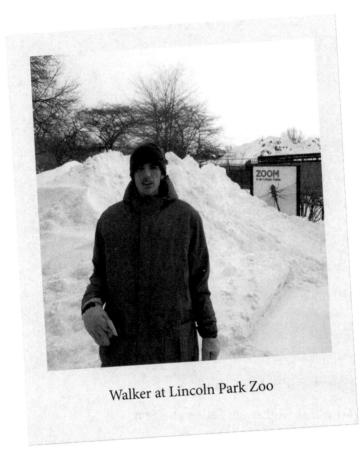

Walker at Lincoln Park Zoo

CHAPTER 1

Zoo–Train–Walk

December 2013

EVEN UNFLAPPABLE ABRAHAM LINCOLN seems to be feeling the chill today. With snow on his head and on his lapels, he looks as if he'd rather hunker down under his big chair than yet again deliver the speech he perpetually does in this lovely setting.

No…wait. That's me who would like to crawl under a chair. My son Walker has been pulling me along rapidly on this dark and late December afternoon before Christmas, and I am very tired and very uncomfortable. For years I've projected my feelings onto this statue, "Standing Lincoln," in Chicago's Lincoln Park. I've passed him hundreds of times and in many moods: worry, happiness, occasional euphoria.

This day my bronze old friend catches me in a time of high anxiety. Walker has what is called "low-functioning" autism, a term that doesn't really help describe him much but does nail down a few key difficulties. At 28, he's a big guy—six foot three—and terrifically good-looking. Monday through Friday he lives in a group home on the North Side and on weekends he stays at his family home with his mother Ellen, his brother Dave, and me.

This Saturday has been a typical one in some ways. I picked him up at the group home at 9 a.m. and we went for a long drive. At noon we hung out in the house, though "hanging out" doesn't capture the tricky, strenuous, tense arrangements we make to manage him. Walker is the most kinetic guy in the world: he never sits still and is always moving and demanding things. In the past it was usually food. These days he has very little appetite and has become worryingly thin but still hasn't slowed down a bit.

This afternoon the cry was, as it always is on Saturday, "Zoo–Train–Walk!" This is his telegraph-speak for "Let's get out and take our long walk, Dad!" His autism mainly manifests itself as a communication problem. He is verbal, but shrinks his few statements into the shortest form possible: "Shoes and socks!" for "Let's get out of here"; "Gurnee Mills!" for "Let's get in the car and take the long drive to Gurnee"; "Fancy Free!" for "Let's watch the YouTube video of Fred Astaire singing and dancing to the Irving Berlin song 'Fancy Free.'"

Yes, autistically, he has trouble communicating. But, un-autistically, he wants to do all these things *with* someone, never alone—never off, in the phrase I've learned to despise, "in a world of his own."

On this cold, cold Saturday in the winter of what the weather sages on TV are calling "the polar vortex," Walker is holding my hand and pulling me along faster than my shaky knees want to go. He stops and shouts "Pen!" This is Walker code for "Let's write down another schedule!" Every statement Walker ever makes must be followed by an exclamation point, inadequate as the punctuation mark is. Laptops don't have a key for "Urgent. I'm afraid the future will disappear if the words aren't in front of me right now. Hurry!"

Although he already has five Dad-printed schedules in his hand, I know better than to insist on reading one of these old, snow-soaked memos again. So we sit down on a bench near the statue and I take the occasion to breathe and think and let my knees throb in peace. I pull an index card out of my back pants pocket and a pen out of a coat pocket and begin naming the notable stops and road markers of the immediate trip ahead: "BF" for the statue of Benjamin Franklin; "BW, ducks geese seagulls, and red-winged blackbird" for the sights we see along the boardwalk over the lagoon, even though I know no self-respecting fauna will appear during our polar vortex.

⟶ ⟵

The first list I printed was at the beginning of our expedition when we got off the subway a mile and a half back from this point. That was where I did my preliminary knee-check—Are my Walgreens knee braces firmly in place? Yes!—and calculated that the old joints would probably hold out. At 64, I've been buffeted a bit by the usual bodily breakdowns, but this knee thing has produced real concern. "Zoo–Train–Walk!" is basic to our father–son relationship. Long hikes through the city practically define us as a team. If I could no longer hack them, a central pleasure of both his and my life would vanish.

Walking fast and far through the city is our big bonding moment. From the time he was a toddler in a stroller, he has delighted in street faces, clerks in stores, ambulances on the street, spectators at the Marathon, marchers in the Pride Parade, crowds at the Air Show, breast cancer walkers in pink, sunbathers on the beach. He has reveled in the change of seasons, the changes in the weather, the sea of humanity in the zoo on a warm day, the privacy of our zoo on frigid days when we're the only visitors there. Throughout our walks, on normal days, his face is lit up with pleasure and his smile never goes away. He looks at the sky as if the parachutes with food rations have finally arrived. He looks at strangers as if they were old friends emerging through the arrivals gate at O'Hare.

And I have learned to see all this through his eyes and learned to appreciate our city pretty much as he does. It's not a subtle thing. It's just an unavoidable effect of being near someone with such deep appreciation of his world. Anyone who catches sight of Walker picks up on it. Speed-walking along, I see the faces of passersby light up with smiles when they spot him. Of course, some of the smiles are reactions to our traveling comedy routine: two tall men holding hands, the leader smiling and tugging behind him an old guy who's trying in vain to keep up.

Unfortunately, this snowy and dark Saturday afternoon is not a normal day. Walker is not grinning, and I am not happy. The staff at his group home say that he's become more and more unmanageable, even dangerous: hitting staff and other clients, becoming "anti-social" and ignoring the other residents, shouting "Mommy Daddy!" at them for no reason, and not eating. So for months now we have tried to minimize his time at the home by picking him up every day after his vocational training at 3 p.m. and bringing him back there only to sleep at night. The sole activity that really relaxes him, that really helps his spirit, is this walk, which I take with him rain, polar vortex, or shine. He rarely smiles now but races determinedly down the street as fast his dad can stand.

→ ←

At the start of our hike near the subway station, we sat and I wrote about the route ahead. The huge Starbucks next to Second City at North and Wells will be our first stop and it will be where I will try hard to get him to eat something. Normally a voracious omnivore, he's developed a maddening aversion to food. He has seen doctors many times over the last year for a variety of reasons, but this eating problem hasn't risen to the alarm levels of a medical emergency. It's just one of the items in the concern overload Ellen and I have been living with of late.

After writing his first schedule on a note card and talking about the weather and what we see on the street, I untangle my iPod headphones to listen to my book. Long ago I learned to augment my pleasure on our walks with books. Audio books have been key therapy for me for years. Driving, speeding down sidewalks with Walker, walking the dog—all have been occasions for me to see for some minutes through someone else's eyes and live mentally in a new place.

I try to be good and choose smart and improving books like *Thinking Fast and Slow* by Daniel Kahneman and *A History of Warfare* by John Keegan. But I mostly listen to activate pleasure centers in the brain. My drug of choice has always been P.G. Wodehouse's Jeeves and Wooster novels. I have listened to all of them many times and always know what's coming, and yet every sentence is still a treat. I like to imagine that I am Jeeves and Walker is Bertie: he needs me and I loyally spring to his aid and his problems are silly, solvable, and calamity-free.

However, for the last week I've been reading a book for sheer inspiration in this season of weather and worries: *Endurance*, the classic history of Ernest Shackleton's abortive Antarctic expedition. As we race-trudge along, I think of heroic Shackleton and his men eating nearly raw seal meat, huddling together at night in soaking clothes against freezing temperatures, straggling across ice floes day after day without hope of rescue. Walker and I are much like them, I think, pushing against the elements and hoping for miracles, persisting despite shaky knees and exhaustion and stress. (The fact that we duck into a Starbucks for a pumpkin spice latte with whipped cream whenever possible just gives our adventure the cozy gloss it needs.) One line from the book especially struck me this week and I rewound it several times and committed it to memory: "Life was reckoned in periods of a few hours, or possibly only a few minutes—an endless succession of trials leading to deliverance from the particular hell of the moment." This sentence seems to symbolically sum up life these days with Walker, at home, out in the street, in his group home, and especially the impossibility of knowing if deliverance is even possible.

⇥ ⇤

As we walk the mile through snow and slush to Starbucks, Walker stops and says "Pen!" several more times and each time I turn off my iPod—often I just give up on it—tuck into a store doorway with him, and write his list of destinations again. Without the hard copy of his itinerary to look at, Walker seems to think the future will go up in smoke, almost as if he were blind and couldn't count on the continuance of the sidewalk ahead. I try strategies to kid him out of this compulsion—the joke, the stern order, the promise of fun to come—but in his current thoroughly rattled state, none of these tactics can work and the "Pen!" stops are sadly frequent. Even now, after years of more or less patiently dealing with his habit of fatal doubt, I can still boil with impatience. But the stars are aligned today and I am on my good behavior. After all, I ask myself, what would Shackleton do?

We cross North Avenue at Wells and approach the corner Starbucks, one of our favorites. Walker loves Starbucks. Even though this one is huge, noisy, and usually crowded, he magically waits in line here, even very long ones, with the nonchalance of the flaneur out on the town. It's where he gets to feel like the young man that he is and not a victim defined by a disability. Pretty women smile at him. Baristas know him and like him and patiently wait for him to give his order. The routine in recent months has been for him to say, so quietly and haltingly as to be inaudible, "Croissant." Servers familiar with him know the secret and breezily retrieve one for him. Novice baristas are baffled: Why the hush-hush? They look at him, quickly take in the two of us, and inevitably smile as I repeat the word.

But none of this happens today.

Right away as we walk in we become the floor show. Walker is agitated, shaking his arms, grabbing me, pushing toward the front of the line, and shouting "Croissant!" as though he expected one to fall into his mouth on command. I try to take off my gloves, hat, and scarf while impossibly helping him with all of his at the same time. The two of us are sweating from the walk and looking like trouble—maybe big trouble—to the people around us. At this point, certain emergency protocols learned from hard experience kick in. My first rule is "Always appear calm and in charge. Smile. No matter how threatening my child appears to people, they will take their cue about the situation from you, the responsible and wise father." Check. So I try this because it normally works—in fact, it worked like a charm in his teen years. But this gets me nowhere. The second rule is "Get the kid out safely and away from people if he can't be calmed down. And keep smiling." Today my performance is not too bad, but no Tony award. I fake calmness and fake mastery of the situation well enough, but actual smiling is beyond my skill set.

→ ←

Outside in the falling snow, we struggle to put our arctic gear back on. All the gloves are accounted for! Yes! (We lose gloves all the time. As a consequence, we always wear the cheapest ones we can find.) Walker instantly calms down. No grin on his face, but no distress either. We manage to get past Walgreens without the old familiar approach-avoidance struggle on his part and mine to go in and buy ice-cream cones. In all weather—just like his father—he can eat ice cream, any amount. Of course, Walgreens is our most frequent stop for treats. There are so many stores in this uber-franchise popping up that a space alien on a quick bus tour would think the city's name must be "Walgreens."

But Walker's strange new aversion to eating wins out. I write another note: "Lincoln Park–Statue of AL–Statue of BF," and we're off. Past the Moody Bible Institute and past the History Museum, he is pulling me through the south end of the park, which looks like a Christmas card here at dusk in the falling snow. But I am cranky. Cold and sweating under my many layers of outer and inner wear, knees aching, and iPod battery running out, I look forward to the Abe Lincoln station stop. We sit on a bench and I write his note about the upcoming route and get my first positive idea of the day: take a picture.

Walker is a little vain—yet another "non-autistic" trait of his—and likes to stop for a photo. His parents have always rained praise on him for his good looks, and, thankfully, he buys it. I have him stand near Honest Abe and once again give him my standard lecture about our fellow Illinoisian and how he struggled against obstacles as a young man. Sometimes it seems to me that Walker understands to the point of boredom everything I say. He can smile and look knowing in such a way that I'm almost embarrassed to be going through my spiel again. So I make an Educated Empathetic Guess about what he'd like to say to me.

Dad, really, another lecture? Yes, I know Abraham Lincoln had a very rough childhood. Yes, I had one too. And normally I like my picture taken. But I want to get going. Sorry about your knees. That's why I've been trying to slow down, because I know your knees hurt. But walking faster calms me down. I feel bad about my life right now but I feel free out here. I know every tree, every garbage can, every dip in the sidewalk, and knowing this is relaxing and reassures me. I want to see how the guy is doing, the one with the shopping cart who sleeps under the viaduct ahead, under the blankets. I want to feel the boardwalk under my feet. I want to see the holiday lights in the zoo. Will they be the same as last year? Let's hurry!

Of course, my guesses about what he is thinking are mainly just shots in the dark. Who knows what anybody else would like to say, even good friends who chatter nonstop? But my guesses have a certain credibility too. As his lifelong valet, his Jeeves, I have an insider's feeling for what is going on in his head. Walker communicates all day. Although he can't converse and doesn't even reliably relay yes and no responses, he is still relentless in his messaging. Reading his body language, facial expressions, movements, laughter, silence, shouting, and constant struggles to verbalize can be quite tricky or flat-out impossible. But trying to read him feels natural and is often successful. It's a habit for me and for Ellen. The more we try, the stronger are the chances for true connection. We know that these guesses could be wildly off the mark. In fact, what we guess on one day might change to a very different guess if we happen to think about the same event later on.

But the real sin is not guessing at all.

→ ←

The sun has set completely now and the boardwalk over the lagoon is very dark—a rare unlit, quiet area in the city. The black stillness only makes the zoo holiday lights in the distance seem more magical. Suddenly, with no warning, Walker erupts with "I want pen!" The "I" in this statement is a recent thing and it drives me crazy. It's a startling, piercing, aggressive "I" that feels like a slap. The "want pen," by contrast, is pronounced quietly and normally. The personal pronoun is the important part of the statement, maybe the only meaningful part of the statement. Ellen and I wonder if he has developed this new habit to get attention at his crowded, busy group home, where we suspect that he is actively disliked by the staff. With seven housemates to compete with, Walker may be trying to insist in a new way. This change in how he asks for things suggests vast, unarticulated dissatisfaction.

I write down a new list, but he insists that I write another. Again I write and again he insists. This means he wants me to come up with his thoughts, his words, but I don't know what they would be. This compulsive loop—write, shout, pull out another index card, write, shout—threatens to nail us to this spot indefinitely. So I sternly, impatiently walk ahead and he, fortunately, snaps out of it. These bouts of compulsive schedule making are understandable to me. I imagine that if I couldn't say what I wanted, I too would probably behave just as Walker does. Putting myself in his place takes me pretty far, but the frigid temperature, my damp shirt, and my aching legs push me in a distinctly un-empathetic direction.

As we enter the zoo, all conflict and obsession are gone. I even get a small smile from him as we look at the Christmas lights and displays. For many years we have taken in these lights, and visions of previous holidays dance in our heads. A loudspeaker blares Nat King Cole but the cold temperature has kept the numbers of zoo walkers down today. The normally crowded cafeteria in the zoo, the midpoint of our trek, is blessedly free of lines today. This is a warm and welcoming place for us. Cashiers Linda and her twin sister Glenda have served Walker French fries and Cokes since he was a toddler and the cafeteria was located in the beautiful Café Brauer building. They've watched him get bigger and bigger and heard my mini-reports about his progress in every season of every year. On busy days, the friendly men who serve us the fries sometimes wave to us over the heads of the multitude as soon as we walk in the door. Like visiting movie stars, we give the long line a miss and pick up our order.

One benefit of our walks through the city is the way micro-communities spontaneously materialize. Wherever we go, our repeated eccentric presence brings smiles and friendly chit-chat. People know Walker's name and ask him how he's doing. I like this very much and especially like the positive charge

Walker very clearly gets from it. He usually doesn't or can't smile at a clerk or server he's come to know when we actually meet, but just afterward a pleased-with-himself smile blooms across his face. He's out in the world, not isolated or trapped. In this way the big anonymous city imitates the intimacy of a small town.

We sit down at a table with his fries and his Pepsi (I heroically don't get these treats for myself but do steal some of his) and listen to "Have Yourself a Merry Little Christmas" coming from a player piano nearby. I start to talk to him about the other times we've shared in just this spot with just this piano playing the same carols.

But today, this is only for a moment.

He jumps up and shouts, "Write stuff down!"—his other phrase for Jeeves, the stenographer—so I throw away the untouched fries and Pepsi—$6.01 but who's counting?—and guide him out the door to a nearby bench where I write down the route ahead. There's another hour plus of walking still to come, another hour which, on better days, would be quite welcome to both of us. But right now, my body aching and the snow falling harder than before and the wind blowing, I'm not what you might call a festive trekker.

After we exit the zoo and approach the corner of Clark and Webster, I start lobbying for the bus. Normally, Walker wants nothing to do with a ride, preferring to dash along with me. I begin, "Do you want to take the bus or walk to Walgreens Number 2?" (All the Hughes Walgreens stores are denominated by numbers.) No answer. I repeat. No answer. This goes on for a few minutes until we reach the corner and he shouts, "Bus!" Ah, I think, deliverance at last! Bob—our brave, courageous, and bold polar explorer who has already eaten his last sled dog and watched the ice floes melt all around him—has been spared at the eleventh hour.

The bus comes quickly and on this blizzardy day is very crowded. Walker is so agitated, however, that people immediately get up and give us two designated "handicapped" seats behind the driver. In the old days, say a year ago, we never would have sat here. We're not handicapped—not us! Walker was only "disabled" to people who bothered to peer at him for a bit. But now in his anxious condition, arms shaking and the shout of "Write stuff down!" hitting people between the eyes at close range, it's definitely a "Let's make way for these two!" situation.

A CTA bus displays humanity at its finest. Sure, there are occasionally some baddies—flashers, stabbers, that sort of folk—but for Walker and me the Chicago commuters are practically saints. This winter, when we've had recourse to the bus more than ever, people smile and eagerly give up their seats, putting themselves sometimes to great inconvenience. As I sit with him and write yet another note card, people smile—not condescendingly or critically or curiously—but just in an appreciative way. Part of the reason is Walker himself. Even in his strangely frightened state, you can tell he's a good guy, a sweet guy. Nobody quizzes me about his problem, although I assume some would like to. There are so many stories in "the naked city," as an old TV cop show used to describe New York, that the occasional zany pair hardly reaches the threshold of surprise.

→ ⟵

Lurching along on the bus, we warm up and I think about the fix Walker and Ellen and I are in right now. (Dave is not currently "in a fix." But in the long run, as his parents age, God only knows.) My head is swimming. When we found a group home for Walker five years ago, we thought we had taken a big and reassuring step. Good group homes are rare and difficult and often impossible to squeeze into in Illinois, which is infamous for being one of the worst states in the country in its care for disabled adults. So when we and other parents helped a small foundation create a fine CILA—a "community integrated living arrangement"—that had a good vocational program, we thought we were, if not sitting pretty, at least breathing easier. The future is the ultimate concern of aging parents of disabled adult children: Our child has friends—us. And knows he is loved—by us. And knows he will be safe and secure—as long we live. But what then?

But the group home and the job program have slowly but quite surely become toxic for Walker. Right now we are looking hard for a new place for him, but our confidence in him has been shaken. Is he, as the staff members at his home repeatedly tell us, a danger to other people? Is he hopeless and actually bottoming out of his vocational program? Does he need some kind of institutional restraint situation, as people at his CILA imply over and over again? If so, would he be thrown out of any program we manage to find?

The gentle, friendly, charismatic Walker I've always known and still know doesn't resemble this violent wild man that he's accused of being. We never see the Mr. Hyde identity that supposedly springs into being when we're not around. But he has changed. His smiles are painfully infrequent. He's high-strung, anxious, too thin, and seems to find no fun in life other than these long walks and drives with me. I have many questions for him that he can't answer: What's wrong? How do you feel about where you live? How do the staff at your house treat you? How do you feel about your housemates? Very simple statements would solve it all: *X is mean to me. My stomach hurts. I'm afraid of Y. The house makes me crazy. Voc is boring. My head hurts. I'm lonely. I'm worried about my future.* Even solid yes and no answers to lobbed questions could solve most of the problems: Do you like your house? *NO!*

But he can't manage this, and therein lies the dire fix he's in. Looking at his face, his handsome, anxious, drawn face, brushed like mine by the winter coats of the commuters jammed together in front of us, I feel my heart breaking with bewilderment at it all. How did he—we—get here? Where is all this heading?

Within a few weeks we would know, when our struggle to restore his true self would become a struggle to save his life.

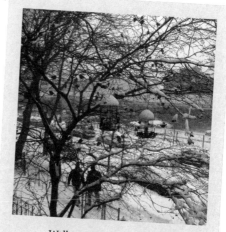

Walker and Dad setting out for Zoo–Train–Walk

CHAPTER 2

"What's Your Plan?"

Winter 2007

"BEAUTIFUL ANIMAL! BEAUTIFUL ANIMAL!"

Our old television friend, Crocodile Hunter Steve Irwin, was shouting in ecstasy as he caressed a big snake he'd just extricated from a tree. The thing looked horrific, as if it carried its own slithering hell with it wherever it went. Holding the snake at the neck while its jaws were open wide, the happy croc hunter was in an altered state of nature worship. Dave, Ellen, and I were glued to our TV screen in howling amazement at the scene. Walker was behind us bouncing on his therapy ball. "One of the deadliest snakes in the world! Look at that jaw! He could tear my face right off! Beautiful animal!" This was too much for the Hugheses.

I said, "Hey, Steve, it's not Miss Universe 2005!"

Ellen said, "So gorgeous! Yes, my first thought as he swallows my arm."

Dave said, "Hey, buddy, it's a snake! It's not Lassie!"

Beat. "I don't need THAT today!" Walker shouted, jumping off his ball, throwing himself on the couch and doubling up with laughter. He looked as if he'd never seen anything so funny in his life.

Dave, Ellen, and I stared at him as he grinned and laughed— and were stunned.

→ ←

This rare, isolated incident stayed vivid in my mind because it contained so much: (1) Walker actually uttering audibly a kind of remark he probably thought often. How much else is he aching to say? (2) Walker showing how much he'd like to be an everyday part of the family conversational world. (3) Walker showing a merry, ironic sense of humor that matched his family's. This precious moment and several others like it became part of the family saga that Ellen and I wanted to keep going. We understood him in a way we believed few could. And we hoped to continue to cultivate a family world that could bring out his nature further as time went by.

But—the biggest "but" of all—we weren't going to live forever. This happy family scene was doomed, at the very least by the passage of time. We needed to think about his adult future without us.

For Ellen and me, the trick question always lying in wait was "What's your plan?" In Walker's teen years this was a frequent question, always uttered with kindly intentions. It was the rhino in the room, the shock coming in the near or less-near future when we would be gone or no longer able to handle him. Ellen or I would be talking on the phone with a friend and chatting away breezily and then, like the Spanish Inquisition in the old Monty Python sketch, The Question would pop up out of nowhere.

What we wanted to say in response was something like "Plan?! We don't have no stinkin' plan!" Of course, the friendly, innocent questioner had no idea she had touched our hypersensitive Nerve of Insanity. And, of course, we always laughed and said something like "Well, the plan is to get through the next day without starting a heroin habit, ha ha."

In truth, our anger came from the fact that we had no plan. Walker was getting older and wiser, we thought, but not improving in the ways of worldly competence. He was still a joy but still difficult and demanding. He could not converse. He could not walk safely alone outdoors (or perhaps he could, but we would never try to discover this). He couldn't work at a job without aid or play a game of any complexity or prepare his own food or wash himself well.

Our early hopes for him breaking through autism's barriers had not materialized. We continued to hope for great things, but we knew we also had to devise a practical stratagem for the future. Our excuse for not doing so—the daily hard work of just living with him and maintaining smiles on our faces— was quite good, if we did say so ourselves. Walker was a happy person, but could he be so once his mother and father were, in the Python phrase, "pushing up the daisies"?

So we did eventually patch together a plan and throw ourselves into it with energy. A foundation was opening up a new adult CILA on Chicago's North Side and we decided to throw ourselves into helping them with energy. I say "we," but Ellen was the real worker here. She networked with influential people, she wrote successful grant proposals, she attended meetings and made friends. She was, as always, our marriage's ambassador to the outside world, the sunny face of "Ellen and Robert." My job was Walker-wrangling and teaching at my college and making sure I eventually earned a pension. Thus I had the harder job—except on the days when Ellen did.

A key advantage to this new CILA was going to be that Pam and Daryl (not their actual names) would be associated with it. Walker already knew Pam as a friend. She had worked with him in the vocational program for five years. She had visited him in the psych ward during one of his lowest points. Daryl and Walker went way back—Daryl had been Walker's teacher since he first attended school at age 11. Daryl knew him well and liked him. These two would be loved figures who could make the home feel familiar from the outset. And they wouldn't be unduly surprised at any typhoons of trouble the switch to a group home might entail.

It was a crucial moment to act. Transitioning from a child group home to an adult one is a no-brainer: when the child reaches 22 in Illinois, the move is automatic. But people like Walker, who have lived in their family's house their whole lives, have a harder time finding a CILA. Because we had friends associated with this foundation and had worked to create the new home, Walker had a good chance—perhaps his only chance—to secure the placement he would eventually need. If we didn't take advantage of this moment, perhaps we would never get another.

→ ←

But all the time we were anxiously working to establish a home for him, we were, of course, anxiously ambivalent about the whole idea of his moving out. It was a searing, devastating, horrible decision for several reasons.

For one thing, we weren't the kind of parents who put our child in a home, for God's sake! Not us! We were autism Hero Parents who could handle anything. We were positive people who were masters of the self-fulfilling prophecy: Walker would keep improving as long as he lived with people who believed in him and predicted success—people like us. Our great achievement, we thought, was the fact that he had maintained his essential character trait through thick and thin: his smile. From the time he was a baby standing in his crib and greeting us in the morning with a 150-watt grin until this moment, when his eyes would gleam as if every walk down the street and every book we read with him was an unbelievable treat, his smile defined him. We hadn't "saved" him from autism, true; we now recognized that he would probably never win a Nobel Prize in physics. But we had created an environment that permitted his best self to thrive, and we were proud of this. Might this end if he lived away from us?

For another, wasn't it possible that Walker could feel abandoned, cut off most of the time from Ellen and me and Dave, his closest friends? Living in a home with other autistic housemates—people who, like him, had great trouble connecting with others—and a staff that might misunderstand him, would he simply despair? We were close to our boy and knew him well, knew how truly normal he was behind autism's screen. We knew how to deal with his "challenging" (one of my favorite euphemisms) behavior and maintain good cheer and loving support. Could the staff at a small group home really treat him well despite the "challenges" he would present?

And we would just plain miss his company. We liked him.

But we also saw advantages, or told ourselves we saw advantages: He might really like the move. Maybe he could think of the place as a fraternity house with friends. Maybe he thought it's squirrely to live with Mom and Dad and be treated like a perpetual child. When I thought of how eagerly I went to live in a college dorm many years before, of how wrapped up I became in my new life and how I never looked back, I imagined that something similar must be—could be?—going on in Walker's head. Perhaps the move would mean a real maturing event in his life, a genuine step forward.

Another advantage was the selfish one: we could breathe a little. We had neglected most of the normal householder things. Our walls hadn't been repainted in 25 years. In fact, our house was literally falling down due to a never-fixed expensive defect in its foundation. We were deeply in debt—although Ellen now had a full-time job, most of Walker's life she had stayed home dealing with his many issues. Our medical bills, even with our insurance, were very high. With Walker living away from us on weekdays, Ellen could work with less stress and I could grade papers without continuous interruption. I'd become accustomed—so much so that the routine had become part of my nervous system—to reading a student's essay in stages: sit, scan, read a half, get up, deal with a Walker issue, sit down, pull myself together, read the rest and hope the comments I proceeded to write made sense. Repeat.

⇥ ⇤

Once the house had been found, there were delays in opening it for the residents. It was a lovely old large place with three floors, gorgeous woodwork, and a big yard, and Walker would have a fine corner bedroom all to himself on the second floor. But the delays were agonizing. It was an anxious winter for Walker; at least we presumed it was. Since Christmas we had been telling him about his big move: he would have a nice room of his own; he would be living with some housemates he already knew from his school; he would be busier and have more fun; and we would take him home every weekend to do all the things we always do. Instead of having just home and school, he would have his vocational training, his own cool apartment with friends, and his home with Mom and Dad. "Life is going to be terrific," we said—convincingly, we hoped. We would tell him all this in a matter-of-fact way, not getting all rah-rah about it, yet not hiding the fact of the big change coming. But he never reacted in any way we could discern to all our talk. As far as he was concerned, judging by his outward behavior, we could only conclude the coming rupture was no big deal to him. Even when, in early March, we finally had a date for the move, he still maintained a flat affect about it.

Someone who didn't know him might say, "Well, of course he doesn't understand what's going on because he doesn't understand language. After all, he can't respond to simple directions like 'Please pick up your shoes and put them in the closet.' How can he comprehend a relatively sophisticated agenda like 'Next week you will move to a new home and see your parents only on the weekends'?" Even Ellen and I were having trouble believing he understood what we were talking about, and we were the great apologists for the idea that there was a normal heart and mind (better than normal, actually) underneath his autistic front. In the popular computer metaphor, autistics have trouble "processing" language, and this certainly seemed true. His brain often seemed overloaded with sensory data and this prevented focus on, say, "Don't get spaghetti sauce all over your shirt!" How, therefore, could Walker comprehend that a global life change was ahead?

But he did comprehend—all too well.

It was four o'clock on the Monday morning before the Wednesday of his big move. Ellen and I woke suddenly in the darkness to the sound of Walker loudly moaning and his rickety daybed in the living room squeaking and rattling spasmodically. Was he having a bad dream? We tumbled down the stairs and found him twitching and shaking and apparently asleep. We shook him and repeated, "Wake up, man! Wake up, Walker!" But we knew, maybe right away, that he was having a seizure, an extremely serious one—the worst since he was five years old.

A fire truck and ambulance arrived within minutes of our calling them, and six or seven giant fire fighters and EMTs stomped reassuringly up our narrow front stairs into the house. Ellen said, "Oh, sorry, I didn't mean to call in a fire truck too!"

One of them said, "Do you want us to leave?"

"God, no!" Ellen said.

It turned out that getting Walker down our long flight of front steps was a four-man job anyway. Big, heavy, and limp, he was no easy lift. Ellen and I had the same thought: Would our flimsy, shaky front steps support all these guys without a further catastrophe? They did! And the inert son and his terrified father went in the ambulance to the nearby hospital emergency room.

⇥ ⇤

Ellen stayed home a few minutes to explain to Dave about what was going on: "Yes, Dave, another Walker emergency."

Now 20, Dave had been living with Walker emergencies for his whole life. He had watched as his older brother flailed through psychotic episodes and seizures and behavior breakdowns of many varieties. He had watched his parents handle all this sometimes well and get happy results, sometimes badly and near-disastrously. A loving and sensitive and observant person, he had watched helplessly as all the king's horses and all the king's men tried and failed again and again to rescue his brother. Now a junior at Columbia College and living at home, he was still experiencing the full sibling-of-a-disabled-child catastrophe: trying to carve out a normal life for himself while surrounded by a troubled brother and troubled parents.

Soon Ellen joined me at the hospital. More level-headed than I was in these circumstances and better able to mentally retrieve crucial information about Walker's medical history, she became, as always, Walker's main medical interpreter. He had taken seizure medications ever since his first big emergency at five, but we wondered if he had been having small seizures—"sleep seizures"—all along during the night. Various attempts had been made to get a sleep EEG, but he had no tolerance for the bonnet of annoying electrodes that had to be worn all night to get reliable results. He would wait, perfectly still, as we painstakingly glued the wires to his head and affixed the bonnet intended to hold the electrodes in place. Then he would put his head on his pillow, and we would get our hopes up. Then five, ten, or 30 minutes later, he would smile and whip them all off in a smooth, impressive Harry Houdini gesture that left us breathless.

Almost as soon as he entered the ER, the doctors determined that the seizure was over. They also said that he was already on the right dose of medication and that this episode was "just one of those things." So later that day we took him home and proceeded to stare at him obsessively through the day, jumping to dire conclusions about his every twitch and eye movement. At night the experience played out again as predictably as some scene in a Muppet tape that Walker liked to rewind perpetually. We all went to bed as on the previous night. We all went to sleep, although this time Ellen and I did a lot of staring at the ceiling and listening. Then near sunrise, once again, the moaning, the squeaking bed, the tortured young man, the frantic parents.

There is nothing quite like the helplessness a parent feels while watching a child's galloping seizure in real time. There is simply nothing to do, except to keep the child safe from injury, pray that this isn't the end, and get medical help fast. We had thought in our naïve way that his seizure era was over, that he had grown out of the problem. But here was the nightmare again. The idea of his "growing out" of things was a necessary survival delusion on our part, entailing this kind of shock sooner or later.

This time, to our relief, the seizure ended and he woke up. So we dispensed with the ambulance and raced with him in the car to the ER. Unfortunately, he was a different patient this time, anxious and awake. Revived and by now used to this seizure routine, he was not particularly happy with being cooped up with his parents in the small examining space. Controlling and pacifying him in the ER or a hospital room demanded more personnel than a mere mother and father. It also required powerful imagination, sunny cheerfulness, and raw muscle power.

The wait was always exacerbated by the Big Tease. Nurses or nurse's aides would pop in from time to time and tell us things to get our hopes up. But we had learned through bitter experience over the years in many hospital visits that statements like "We'll soon have a room to admit Walker to the hospital" were composed of English words all right, but they carried very little actual meaning. In fact, the more specific the statement— "A room should be ready in an hour"—the more vaporous the promise. "An hour" could mean two, three, or eight hours. Getting a room "ready" seemed to be a special task for the Army Corps of Engineers. The all-time whopper, the nastiest desert mirage was this one: "The nurse will be here shortly with the discharge forms." These words really meant "Abandon hope, all ye who have entered here."

This time was no exception. We wrote list after list for him, promising all kinds of great treats and trips for him at the end. We physically restrained him when he tried to get away. Things were transpiring in this familiar turbulent way when we were interrupted by an uplifting little miracle. Suddenly, a hand pulled the curtain aside, and there appeared our family physician, Dr. Frank Weschler, who happened to be making his hospital rounds at that moment. He was very well liked by Walker, who regarded every trip to his office—really, it is not too strong to say this—the way a toddler might regard a trip to see a department-store Santa Claus. "Hi, Walker!" the doctor said, stepping forward to where Walker was sitting.

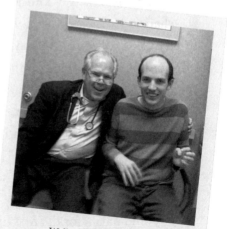

Walker and Dr. Weschler

Walker reached out, grabbed Frank's hands, and placed them on each of his own shoulders, as if to say, "Doctor, heal me!" All of us, doctor included, were awestruck. I think our minds were spinning with the things that this gesture of our "nonverbal" autistic young man suggested: deep trust and hope, strong personal connection, and tremendous anxiety. From time to time, all his life, Walker surprised us with these moments of clear, powerfully telegraphed emotion—unmistakable signs of his feelings for the people in his life.

Later that day Ellen and I were in the hospital room waiting for his test results. As the hours crawled by, we had the challenge of keeping our six-foot-three linebacker-like son in the room. Barricading the door with a chair, writing lists, singing songs, sneaking in treats, holding him down the best we could, all we could think was "Is this guy ready to live in a group home? How could he be? Are we making a big mistake in sending him there?"

Finally, finally, a knock on the door and I got up from my chair to let the doctor in. He was a different neurologist from the one on the previous day, an older man who seemed to speak from deep experience of this kind of situation. He too told us that the medication was right, that it was just what he would have prescribed for Walker.

"What else is going on in his life? Is there any reason he might be anxious or upset?" he asked us.

"Well," Ellen said, "he's scheduled to enter a group home tomorrow for the first time."

"You mean, for the first time in his life?"

"Yes. He's always lived at home with us. Do you think we might be doing the wrong thing in sending him to live there?"

"Well, if you want him to stop having seizures, get him into that home right away. He's traumatized about the unknown. When he knows what he's really facing, he'll calm down and stop seizing."

Well, duh, Mr. and Mrs. Hughes! We wanted to shake his hand. Everything fell into place for us with that answer. We were doing the right thing. Walker's seizures were based on feelings, on the terror he felt about the future. He *did* understand what we had been talking about for so long. But he couldn't discuss his fright, couldn't verbalize a thing about it. The seizures weren't just "one of those things that happen to autistics." They had a real emotional basis, and a real cure. Beyond the realization that we were doing the right thing, we learned another lesson, one that, unfortunately, we had to relearn again and again in the coming years: Walker understands language much better than he seems. Don't be fooled by his often nonreactive silence when you talk to him.

He gets it.

→ ←

The next day, a Wednesday, was our D-Day, our moment of truth. After Walker's vocational training, we had dinner and watched a movie with him. (Dinner: "spaghetti something else"—cooked noodles, butter and parmesan cheese; movie: *Indiana Jones and the Last Crusade*—20th, 30th time?) Because his new bedroom was already stocked with clothes and a big bed, a boom box, and a large therapy ball to bounce on and decorated with posters, there weren't any more preparations for us. That is to say, there weren't any more healthy busy-work distractions for us. So we three got in the car and drove the 20 minutes to his new home.

Our first worry—whether he would even get out of the car when we arrived—was over in a flash. He walked right up the stairs and through the front door. We walked in behind him and started chatting away merrily with the staff and Walker about the great, activity-packed, wonderful life ahead for him. Then when we turned around to leave, our second worry— whether Walker would tolerate us walking away without him— came true like a blow to the solar plexus. While staff members restrained him, we shut the door behind us and hurried back to the car, listening to his shouts of "Mommy Daddy! Mommy Daddy!"

As we drove away, our third worry—that we wouldn't be able to stand it, that our hearts would be too broken to go on— turned out to be false. Our hearts weren't broken, exactly. We were just stunned, our heads spinning with guilt and betrayal. Sitting in silence, I trusted to the automatic driver part of my brain to make the car go, slow down, turn, stop, speed up. So this was where all our love and "intelligent" parenting had led: to us dropping him off with other people. We felt as if we'd left Granny out on the ice to get her out of the way.

And I couldn't get it out of my head that I'd just betrayed my friend.

We had striven mightily to tell ourselves that this was going to be no big deal. Walker was like a young college student eager to get away from his parents and start adult life. His new home would be like a fraternity house. We were like parents who drop their child off at college, and the kid can't wait for embarrassing Mom and Dad to leave so he can begin the serious business of making friends in the dorm. But all these rationalizations didn't account for our emotional state, our immediate reality; lucky novice empty nesters don't drive away with their child's cry of "Mommy Daddy!" ringing in their ears. So I drove on in the spirit of a hit country song both Walker and Dave loved from that year: "If You're Going Through Hell Keep on Going." We would go on, but this really was hell.

Ten minutes into our silent, slow drive home, Ellen got a call on her cell phone. It was Pam telling her not to worry, that Walker had already calmed down and was smiling and looking forward to the rest of the evening. This was reassuring and we started to breathe a bit more normally. We were grateful to her for understanding so well what we needed to hear at that moment. But our fears were still pounding in our heads: What if Walker just bombs out? What if he is not a match for this home and is considered too much to handle? What if he simply hates the place and hates us for leaving him there?

⟶ ⟻

Later that night, as we sat with unseeing eyes on the couch pretending to watch a second rerun in a row of *Law and Order*, we got another call. A staff member asked, "How do you give Walker a shower in the evening?"

"Why?" Ellen asked.

"Well, right now he's naked and all soapy and singing and bouncing on his ball in his bedroom."

"No," Ellen said, "that isn't part of our normal routine here." They both started laughing.

"It's no big deal," the staff member reassured her. "We were helping him with his shower and he suddenly took off. He's probably thrown by the situation—being naked in front of strangers and all. It's no big deal. It's nothing at all really. Just wondering if you had a hint."

Ellen thanked her for calling and hung up, hintless but relieved. The staff was wise and good humored and saw what a good-natured fellow Walker was.

We thought, *This just might work. It just might work.*

CHAPTER 3

A Brave New World

AND IT DID WORK.

Walker's first days in his new home were unbelievable. That is to say, Ellen and I couldn't believe things were going well. The staff at the home—with good cheer, intelligence, and empathy—was making sure this radical transition went smoothly. Walker had never spent a night away from home, except for hospital visits. And his recent seizures could easily be seen as a sort of whole-body rejection of this group-home idea. The big move was necessary, we knew, but was it possible?

His first night was a Wednesday. Thursday night came and no late-night call from the CILA. Friday night and, again, no call. Ellen and I were breathing almost normally by this time, but—worrying being a kind of lifestyle for us—we were already focused on the next big test: the weekend. We were expected to take him home Saturday and Sunday. It seemed to us premature to do this even briefly when he was just getting used to his new digs. But a founding principle of the CILA was that the client would spend every weekend with his parents to keep up that family connection. As helicopter parents extraordinaire, we heartily endorsed this idea. As dedicated worriers, we dreaded what might happen that weekend.

Sure, we knew that we could pick him up as planned on Saturday morning. Sure, we knew he'd eagerly get in the car and do all his normal at-home stuff. But would he go back on Sunday night?

This was the Big Question. We had learned long ago that you can't really "make" a child get out of a car and walk into a building, even a small child. When Dave was in the throes of OCD fears in the third grade, we couldn't get him dressed in the morning, much less abduct him and deliver him to school. Unless you're willing to shackle the child, put duct tape over his mouth, carry him over thresholds, and lock him into rooms, you can't make a move. When the child is, like Walker, six foot three and 180 pounds, abduction is alarmingly bad thinking.

Because of Walker's silence, we had no real clue about what was ahead.

→ ←

That weekend, then, was nominally a normal one—Hughes normal. We three got into the Dodge Caravan to drive to the Gurnee Mills mall. Now, for what some in the autism community call "neurotypical" families, a trip to the Gurnee Mills mall from Chicago would be a special consumer event, not something to undertake lightly. It might be a Christmas shopping trek, or a chance to hit an advertised sale at an outlet store. Over an hour's drive away, this was not a place to idly window-shop. But in dozens and dozens of trips to this mall, and the burning of vast quantities of precious fossil fuels and dollars, the Hugheses never bought a thing—that is, never bought a thing other than food. It was, first, an excuse to drive—one of Walker's favorite relaxing activities. Second, it was a means to get out in public.

"Let's get out with the people!" was one of my catchphrases, repeated before every excursion.

I always said this enthusiastically but I only half meant it. As a driver, I fought misanthropy mile by mile. My long-suffering family knew well my basic principle of driving: Dad is perfect; other drivers are sociopaths. A driver with my temperamental infirmity is hard to take, and I often wondered what Walker thought as he sat helplessly with his short-tempered dad. He would look interestedly out the window at all times and seemed to pay close attention to the vehicles racing all around us. At every merging traffic entrance, he'd spin around in his seat to check the traffic coming up on the right. Sitting in the front seat, he'd check the side-view mirror for cars behind. I often wondered what he was thinking.

Dad, take it easy! You gotta check your blind spot better than that when you switch lanes. That was a close call but it wasn't that guy's fault. It's not enough to just check your mirror and signal. You have to look. I wish I could show you how to do it. I think I could drive a lot better than you. But don't get me wrong. I like driving with you and Mom. I like to listen to you and Mom make dumb jokes all the time and be happy. I think you're a little too critical of other people, though. And I really hate it when you talk about me like I'm not even here. That really burns me up sometimes.

But being a passenger is great. I like that nobody asks me too many questions when I'm in the car. It's peaceful. I get to think about life—my life and the people in it. I can let my thoughts roam freely. Questions make me nervous. Dad, you're always asking me, "How you doin', Walker? What's on your mind?" I get jittery every time you do that. Don't get me wrong here. I want you to talk to me and really don't like being ignored. I'm a person too and part of the scene, and it's very good to be included. But I feel like I fail every time I'm asked a question. I just can't find the words quick enough. And the longer I look for them, the more I freeze up. I have a lot to say, believe me, but the words just don't come. When I do think of the right word, you and Mom always make such a big deal out of it, like you just won a million dollars. That's nice, but it just builds the pressure and I freeze up even more. If you could just relax, I think I could relax more too.

Imagining what he might be thinking would straighten me out for a while. But bad habits die hard.

Still, driving had another side, a happy one. Just knowing that Walker was relaxed was better than Prozac for us (and some actual pharmaceutical equivalent of Prozac was a daily ritual for all of us). It was a chance to talk and think. We'd drink coffee, listen to music, and chat, usually without interruption. A number of times Ellen and I would get so distracted by our own scintillating conversation that we'd miss an exit. Walker, the living GPS device in the car, would start making a fuss shortly before we needed to turn off. He'd make more noise and even lean forward to grab me by the shoulder. Irritated, we'd sharply tell him to sit back and be quiet. Only minutes later, speeding past the exit, would we realize what his fuss was all about.

And driving alone with Walker on the weekend was usually very pleasant. I would listen to my downloaded audio books—one after another after another—and he would listen to country music on the radio. One of the odd pleasures of the books was the fascinating effect they had on the landscape we drove through. Simply picturing the world of a book while looking at my world created a strange mental superimposition of the author's world on to my streets, my shopping malls, my forest preserves. Ludicrously clashing landscapes only seemed to enhance this effect. I could look out at the rows of mini-mansions near Libertyville and associate them with the rolling green hills and stone fences of James Herriot's *All Creatures Great and Small*. I could drive down Crawford Avenue in Skokie and associate the flat suburb with the Himalayas of Jon Krakauer's *Into Thin Air*. Thus no car trip was mere repetition. Dad was never bored, and the look on Walker's face said that he was quite happy.

This particular Saturday trip was no exception to our Happy Travelers routine. What might happen on the Sunday-evening return to the CILA loomed but didn't crush our spirits. Walker this time was sitting in the front seat, smiling—as was his wont. I'd repeatedly glance to my side at him, pick up his grin, pass it to Ellen in the back seat, where she would reflect it back at me in our frequent, familiar, fun house-of-mirrors-in-the-car effect.

It had not been forever thus. The passenger-side door, for example, was still covered in old duct tape on the chance that Walker might open it at 65 m.p.h. We'd gone through a period two years before when Walker, unaccountably, would get a wild look in his eyes, shout something that sounded like "parmesan shining!" and open the door to get out as I dropped my coffee, grabbed his shoulder, slowed down, and pulled over to the side, all the time shouting at him like a maniac. Putting him in the back seat where there was a child safety lock on the door only delayed catastrophe. More than once he climbed into the front seat and lurched to the door to open it—twice climbing over Ellen. This sudden unpredictable fright of his happened rarely, but it made us wonder for a time if driving with him was out of the question. The possibility of the geography of our lives shrinking in this way was horrible to contemplate.

The passenger's side door had no child lock—the GM designers had not taken into account the Walker Hughes contingency. Duct tape over just the door handle, we discovered, only slowed him a bit; he could pull it all off in what seemed like one swift movement. Duct tape over the entire door, however, slowed him enough for me to pull over and allow him and any other occupants of the car to decompress. (Of course, whatever the solution, it had to involve duct tape, my small brain's range of solutions extending only so far. I'd let duct tape drive the car if I could.) Explaining all this to a passenger unacquainted with the reason for the tape made us sound like lunatics. "Sorry, you can't open the door," we'd say as we arrived at a destination. "I'll come around the car and open it for you."

We never knew what caused these explosions. Small seizures? Sudden real panic? Or what "parmesan shining" meant. Did he see something, some bright overpowering image in his brain? Did whatever it was look to him like shaken parmesan cheese falling in front of his eyes? What other words or combination of words sounded like "parmesan"? Was this an attempt to explain a feature of a seizure? Was I, the driver, somehow the cause—something I was doing or not doing? Ellen and I in our post-mortems of the event would try to reconstruct the context but never came up with anything convincing. Again, the language issue loomed. Whatever was happening, frustration with his inability to express his terror in words, to share his feeling with another person, was a big part of it. Aggressive-looking movements always had behind them fright or frustration. Talking calms people down, but talking was not possible for him.

→ ←

We three got to the mall and started to walk, lurching from one wonderful franchise of deliciousness to the next. Gurnee Mills is unbelievably vast. To navigate properly, one should first imprint on the mind a mental map of the place. It always seemed to me that from the air it must look like one of those police chalk drawings of a splayed-out murder victim. One arm of stores goes north, one leg goes west, and so forth. To Walker it seemed like paradise: loud, full of people, and bulging with junk food emporiums—a site that seemed to invite fast, fun walking and short gourmandizing stops. We'd race down one leg of stores and into Taco Bell for a Cheesy Gordita Crunch, then hike awhile and down another leg to Cinnabon.

This route was similar to our old Field Museum trajectory years ago, now abandoned. Exhibits were to be raced past in predetermined routes on two floors, culminating in the grandest anthropological exhibit of them all, McDonald's, at the lower level. To Walker, the mall seemed little different from a museum: a colorful, fascinating place full of people to see and hear, stuff on exhibit, space to fly through, and food to eat. Of course, it made sense in a way. A mall really is a kind of living museum of the Way We Live Now: shopping is what we do.

We knew these trips were both good and bad for him. The bad was the eating—a terrible indulgence and toxic habit, but not all that different from the way "normal" Mom and Dad ate. The good, however, was incontrovertible. It was an offshoot of our early attempts to teach him greed. When he was three, four, five, we were alarmed at his complete indifference to material things. It wasn't normal, it wasn't American, to not want stuff! Sitting in the shopping cart at Toys R Us, he would barely look at the shiny trucks, the Spiderman action figures, glorious colorful plastic creations of all sorts that we would pass. I'd show him a picture book that talked, something he loved at home, but he wouldn't try to get me to buy it. Never did we experience with him the classic parent nightmare of leaving a store with a screaming kid angry at not getting the toy he wanted. One neurologist early on told us he was "object-oriented." This was the direct opposite of the people-directed boy we knew.

But he did love the store. He loved being with his parents and moving. He loved getting out and looking at people. We called him our "little Ronald Reagan"; like a happy politician, he gorged on eye contact with strangers, enjoyed winning them over with smiles. So we took him out and walked, drove, dived into public places. We explored neighborhoods, walked through the Loop, rode trains just to look out windows at the passing scene. We admired him for his adventure-seeking, citizen-of-the-world identity and we patted ourselves on the back for doing something right. Self-applause, we learned, was as important as self-criticism. Celebrating small successes built confidence; pummeling ourselves for our frequent failures with him easily spiraled into despair.

→ ←

Getting home, we walked up the back stairs into the house, the two-story in the Lakeview neighborhood we call home, Walker in the lead. Dave was in his hideaway, his bedroom, writing, writing, writing. A senior in high school graduating in eight weeks, he lived very much in his own creative head. The writer's knack for storytelling was, in him, like some kind of propulsive force. A successful student, his main work had always been outside of class, writing plays, comic books, sitcoms, short stories, long fiction, songs, mini-musicals, short films. He had fans online, one of them commenting on a comic strip of his, "Any day I get up and I see a new post from Dave Hughes is a good day."

As Walker stomped past the closed door to Dave's cave, Ellen shouted, "Hi, Dave!"

He opened his door and said, "Hi, you guys. Hi, Walker. How'd it go?"

"OK," I said. "Walker's been happy. The test will be tomorrow when we bring him back, I guess."

"How you doing?"

"Just fine," I said. For Dave, a perennial habit was taking all our temperatures in this way. The various answers to "How you doing?" might mean the difference between a relatively peaceful evening and a bumpy one.

"How's your writing going?" Ellen said.

"Good. Good. I started a new comic. I'll tell you about it later."

He then ducked back into his room, and we didn't see him for another couple of hours. His room was a good place to write but also his safe house, his in-home escape from home and the tension of living with stressed-out parents and a troublesome brother. People often asked us, "How do Walker and Dave get along?" I suspected they were hoping for a feel-good story about some kind of odd, magical rapport between them, the kind of story you might catch on a prime-time television special about autism in a family. None existed. Day in, day out, our household always maintained a certain level of tension, for Walker presented, quite literally, minute-by-minute challenges. Dave had lived in this tense environment and vibrated along with it all his life. He'd watched helplessly as his parents tried with only mixed success to handle the antics of his older brother. He had tried and still did try to connect with Walker in one way or another, but his efforts had never succeeded in tangible ways.

→ ←

Entering our house with Walker this day and every day was a *loud* experience. Heavy and hurrying, he'd cheerfully stomp from the back of the house to the front closet and begin, with a smile, to demand spaghetti or a video or a puzzle. Ellen and I would scramble to deal with him while changing clothes, putting away groceries, sorting through mail, or doing the dozens of small tasks that entered the multitasking maelstrom. Our unit was the second floor; our tenant Allan lived on the first. A kind and considerate guy, almost a member of the family, Allan never said anything about the thunder he heard above him through the thin layers of floor and ceiling. Having worked with a friend many years ago to gut this building and put it back together again, I knew how thin this layer was. It had an almost drum-like quality. Allan heard family turmoil, family happiness, family nonsense, high-volume Disney videotapes, and late-night TV talk shows without mentioning his almost certain irritation even once.

The daily storm of our house was more than loud; it was urgent. Everything for Walker had to happen soon, real soon— even better, five minutes ago. The food, the fun, the outing, the shower, the movie—all had to happen now, not later. If grilled cheese sandwiches for four were being made, Walker might say "Grilled cheese!" over and over while they were on the stove, as though he thought parents had some sort of sizzling superpowers. "Wait, Walker. Just wait," we'd hiss or shout or whisper or tease back at him. When the sandwiches had been distributed and everybody, including the cook, was poised to take a bite, Walker would already be done with his and on to the dessert: "Ice cream!" It was a level of tension that we had lived with for many years without entirely accepting it.

What helped to make the tension bearable was the laughter. There was always an edge of teasing to the demands. Usually accompanied by a smile, the repeated demand "Grilled cheese! I want grilled cheese!" seemed like a joke—a very tired one, but still a joke. His face beamed with good nature, even during some exasperating, pushy performances. It was as though a very charming trumpeter was blasting a note from three feet away every few seconds. But without tactics to control his habit and to control our own reactions, our heads were in danger of popping off, as they sometimes did.

On this late afternoon, his cry was "Spaghetti! Spaghetti!" My chosen tactic was Iron Resolution, which involved cooking timers. Some people, perhaps English majors, measure out their lives with coffee spoons, but we Hugheses measured them out with Walgreens $4.99 cooking timers. These little gadgets were all over the house—some broken, some in need of a battery (never to be replaced), some lost and only to be rediscovered on searches for keys or the TV remote control. All of them beeped at a maddening volume just below audible to me, with my geezerish hearing inability.

I stood in front of the stove in the cook's position. Walker took up his post just on the other side of the stove, facing me from his bunker, our dining room. I'd fill a pan with water, turn on the burner, and say, "OK, man. It will take about five minutes for this to boil." Then, with a flourish and a grin, I set a timer for five minutes.

In about 30 seconds, Walker shouted: "Spaghetti!"

"OK, man," I said, quietly and evenly, "gotta start all over again." Then, with another flourish—flourishes are a talent of mine—I poured it out and filled it up, then set the timer again. "Here we go. Five minutes."

Walker stood there, approach-avoidance written all over his face. Yes, he had to say it again. But no, saying it again would delay spaghetti even longer. And delayed spaghetti meant delayed *everything*, all the items on The Schedule for the rest of the evening, all the items that *must* be ticked off. It was much more a schedule issue than a hunger one.

After three minutes, again, "Spaghetti!"

"Sorry, man," I said. "See, the water isn't boiling and we have to start over again. And this causes further delay." Then I poured out, filled up, set the timer, and I heard my own unfamiliarly quiet, even voice saying, "Another five minutes. Don't do it again, Walker."

This routine worked well, on this and on other occasions when my head happened to be screwed on right. Walker followed the timers with good humor for his spaghetti dinner and through this Saturday evening for puzzles, videos, TV programs, shower time, bed. This strategy had been a hard-won victory some years ago. There had been instances when I poured out the boiling water from the pan as often as 11 times—

even tossed the nearly cooked spaghetti noodles—because he couldn't adhere to the regimen.

This kind of rigid, whistle-blowing, dog-training-like stuff ran counter to the parenting style Ellen and I had—if we did indeed have something as grand as a "parenting style." Both of us grew up in loose-discipline homes where we were free to go about the cabin at leisure and didn't "do chores." We had been nice kids, we'd pitched in, and we'd grown up to be respectable voting Americans. We were strongly averse to anything that could be described as "stern." But this timer-orientation, strict or not, cooled off family freneticism and made the house livable.

→ ←

The next day, Sunday, went swimmingly. Walker was happy and so were we. We went on excursions to the forest preserve and our usual big-box stores, but only one question loomed larger and larger as the minutes ticked by: Would he go back?

This was a young man who had lived in his family home all his life. He had much less experience of the world outside than others his age. We had homeschooled him until age 11 because we couldn't find a suitable place for him. He had spent only one night away from home: at a camp for children with disabilities in which he stayed awake the entire night agitating for "Mommy Daddy." When we picked him up the next morning, both he and his saintly, long-suffering personal camp counselor had the wild look of college students who had pulled an all-nighter guzzling coffee before the final exam. What was Walker really thinking about the prospect of calling this CILA his new home? Was his three-night experience thus far just a lark for him? Did he realize what he was actually getting into?

We drove up to the front of his house early that evening and glanced at him in the back seat. He was—yes—smiling! We stepped out of the car and he raced to the door ahead of us, smiling. Then he actually went *through the door* to high fives from the staff.

What's this? we thought, relieved and amazed.

The start of a brave new world?

CHAPTER 4

The Empty Nesters

ELLEN AND I WERE sitting on the couch and watching TV but not focusing on Letterman's monologue very well. Imaginary sights and sounds kept distracting us. A phantom young man kept walking toward the TV, waving his arms rapidly, and smiling, sending the message, *Hey, you guys, pay attention to me.* As we ate chips and salsa, this same phantom would shout *Popcorn party!* from behind us at the dinner table. Down the hall would come the sound of a door closing. I'd think for a split second, *I better check on him.* It was a reflex. We were technically in a relaxed and lounging position, but our senses were still on alert to the son who wasn't there.

Ellen and I had just partially entered the stage called "empty nest syndrome," but the syndrome felt more like a nervous disorder. Sure, we told ourselves, Walker was safe, in good hands, and apparently happy. But a normal American family nest didn't operate like ours. Normal nests don't live and breathe for one increasingly big bird. They don't take their emotional and logistical cues, moment by moment, year after year, from number-one chick. The whole family vibrated with the needs of the charming but demanding Young Master.

For all of his 22 years, we always knew exactly where he was and what he was doing. The toddlerhood stage had never ended in any real sense. One of us was always "on duty"—that is, helping him with eating, the bathroom, his clothes, or being an active teacher and friend. Walker was not a self-starter or even a self-continuer. He always needed to be doing something, and he always needed direction. Even when watching a video, he required a companion-reactor. If he was doing a puzzle, he depended on a companion-hunter for pieces. Walker was, from a narrow parent-monopolizing vantage point, like a whirling, unstoppable, perpetual toddler.

While he was occupied, the other parent would be trying to get something—anything—done. Shop, clean, fix, write, grade, take a shower, go to work, and, oh, actually be a parent to his brother Dave. Everything about our nest was half tended to and looked it. As a bachelor in 1983, I had teamed with a friend to gut and renovate the house. It had been a sorry, half-burned-out building with gang graffiti on the walls. When we were finished, the place looked quite nice: an apartment on the first floor for a tenant, a pleasant apartment above for me and my just-met and married wife, Ellen. It had a fireplace, a high arched ceiling, a fashionable mezzanine bedroom overlooking the living room. It also had an unfinished back porch room, a perpetually leaking roof, and no carpets—but all that, we said, was interesting potential.

But the potential never materialized. The walls were painted in 1983, but 30 years on had never been repainted. The stairs were still bare pine boards. The back porch room—an interesting "space" that seemed ripe for creative home-decorating ideas for starry-eyed Ellen and Bob in 1983—was, by 2007, frightening in its jungle tangle of accumulated family stuff. As homeowners, we looked back to about 1988 as the icy peak of our middle-class normality.

The reason for this poor home-maintenance performance was autism. Medical bills—even after insurance payments—were very high. Trips to the emergency room, hospital psych ward stays, medications, trial therapies, tutors, and private classes cut sharply into our one-parent, English-teacher income. Time was another big factor. Walker was the high-maintenance priority. So house cleaning became quick surface touch-ups. Home repair became a duct-tape and Gorilla Glue expo. Preparations for the rare visitor or Christmas party became a study in home fakery that would make a crooked real estate salesperson blush. Our one financial boon, oddly enough, was not the house but the "location, location, location" it sat on. Our street near Wrigley Field was relatively valuable. "You're sitting on a gold mine," people told us. So the gold mine was mortgaged again and again and again and scheduled to be paid off in our 130s.

→ ←

One spot encapsulated our way of life. Walker had a station in the corner of our dining area—his command post. Here he was never still, always moving, always active. If he turned to his left, he faced our tiny kitchen over a small, low-slung dividing wall. If he faced forward, he could see the TV and everything going on in the living room. If he turned right, he could plunge into his domain: our dining-room table—the oak surface of his home education, his meals, his puzzles, his computer, his books, his boom box. From here he could jump, shout, cajole, joke, laugh, bounce on a therapy ball, and attempt to communicate with us in every way he possibly could. From here he could harass and sometimes help the cook; he could command the TV and videos; he could lobby for treats, for car trips, for long walks through the city. It was the spot of fun, discipline, illumination, entertainment, and frequent nervous breakdowns for all four of us.

He almost never sat. He manned his little station while jumping up and down, bouncing on a therapy ball, or shifting from foot to foot in a stationary rhythmic dance that never varied. His hyperkinetic "sitting" involved such gyrations that our first table and set of chairs had been pummeled, broken, fixed and refixed over the years until finally replaced. In his adulthood, while no master of deportment, he had more of a live-and-let-live attitude toward furniture. His antics were especially hard on the short plasterboard dividing wall between him and the kitchen. We had painted and repainted and repaired this little wall until we gave up and nailed a large white rectangular piece of plastic across it. At first we were proud of our plastic rectangle; like the duct tape crisscrossing cabinets and furniture, we told ourselves it was a clever solution noticed only by pathological fans of home improvement TV programs. As time went by, however, it became just one more weird dark place we no longer really *saw* anymore. We had lived with our patched, disintegrating, unfinished house for so long that we tended to notice it only when a new visitor stopped by. Only then did we imagine what they must be thinking: *How can these people live this way?*

⇥ ⇤

The obvious purpose of Walker's command post was to keep everybody thinking about him, noticing him, forced to interact with him. From here he contradicted, every minute of his life, one of the most popular pieces of conventional wisdom about autism: that autistic people prefer to be alone. A good expression of this idea occurs in the bestselling novel *The Curious Incident of the Dog in the Night-Time.* Here the young autistic protagonist describes his fantasy of a "Dream Come True": to be an astronaut alone traveling in a spaceship. Here, he says, "I wouldn't be homesick at all because I'd be surrounded by lots of the things that I like, which are machines and computers and outer space. And I would be able to look out of a little window in the spacecraft and know that there was no one else near me for thousands and thousands of miles…"

But to our autistic son this dream would be a flat-out nightmare. He never spent time alone. There had been many moments when we would have loved for him to occupy himself in a spaceship of his imagination or upstairs in our bedroom or even in the horrible-but-fascinating-to-a-kid back porch room. But no, he was so far from doing this that he seldom stepped out of our sight. He was a person aching to connect with other persons, to join the social game, if anybody could figure out how to help him. He was a kind of connection freak: sometimes it seemed that if he could talk, he would say continuously from morning to bedtime, "Look at me. Think about me. Pay attention to me, damn it!"

Knowing Walker as we did, Ellen and I worried that one consequence of this autistic-people-shun-company idea would be that teachers, caregivers, potential friends would stop trying to connect. Worse, they would be likely to misinterpret his wild, flailing attempts to communicate as behavior issues. Why work hard to bond with somebody presumed to want nothing to do with you? And how thick-skinned and amazingly determined does a potential friend have to be to keep trying, day in and day out?

This was why we had kept him out of the public school special education system when he was very young—we didn't want him to be isolated in what was, in those years, essentially custodial care. Instead, we homeschooled him in every way we knew how: private lessons, trial therapies, and active, persistent, upbeat attention. Ellen gave up her job at a public relations firm, and I arranged my teaching schedule to be able to spend more time with him. Finally, when he was 11, we found a good school for him that treated him as an individual and not a stereotype. His teachers were insistent on teaching the guy they saw in front of them and not a textbook autistic.

When he came home from school each day, Ellen and I would spring into action again: attempting to homeschool him as far as we could, taking him out for long—we hoped educational—walks through the city. We couldn't conceive of Walker's very existence without our intervention, our interpreting voices. As someone who could not speak for himself, he needed a translator-shadow figure at his elbow. At least this was how we were accustomed to see his interactions with others. We were perpetual interveners, interpreting him before the misinterpretations set in. Anybody who knew us could predict that we would be bad candidates for handling empty nest syndrome gracefully.

A small but classic example of a misinterpretation was "lack of eye contact," a term beloved by teachers and to them suggestive of all manner of trouble. Evaluators in fact often counted the number of times he made eye contact with them within a set number of minutes, as though there were a magic ratio, a tipping point, an "ah-ha!" number, that could predict the winners and losers in school and in life. But we knew his "eye contact" habits were complex and interesting: He could turn away from a steam locomotive or a well-loved aunt, just because he was so thrilled. He could also, unaccountably, stare and stare into the eyes of a person he knew and liked, or just an acquaintance that he wanted to win over. He could look intently at a book we were reading together or turn away inexplicably. He could glance at us with the charm of George Clooney, or share a joke with a sparkling look of total hilarity, but he could also keep his eyes frustratingly averted. Often Ellen and I were certain we knew what was on his mind; other times we hadn't a clue.

But we never had the dead certainty of a teacher armed with a grad school textbook and a few generalizations about autism.

So as empty nesters we were totally at a loss, with no idea how to function without our normal occupation. We wanted to *be there*—to help, to explain, to reassure, to encourage—but we were now cut off, at least until the weekend when we'd pick him up again. For the first time in his life, we had to take the word of other people who were spending more time with him than we were. If they said he did such-and-such, we'd have to take their word for it. If they interpreted his motive in causing some trouble, we had no way of disputing the story. Their witness was all we had now, for Walker was a non-talker. You could accuse him to his face of robbing a bank—he wouldn't contradict you. He might understand what you were saying—we were often not really sure—but he certainly couldn't deny it.

→ ←

So the four of us became three with the remaining chick, Dave, very much still at home with us. Through the years he had developed ways to cope with the wild brother and the upset parents, the main one being to shut himself up alone in his room. By doing so, he was also opening himself up to the wide world via the internet and a wide-screen Macintosh. Always a storyteller, here he wrote like a man on fire: plays, fanfics, parodies, poetry, music. He had tried and tried as a young kid to connect with his big brother, but nothing seemed to work. If anything, he grew to pity his parents and his brother because he could see the fix we were all in. He also rightfully pitied himself, for he knew quite well what he was missing out on. Walker was tall and handsome and two years older than he—a big brother who could have been a cool-guy guide while growing up, helping him to pave his way through school and the social world.

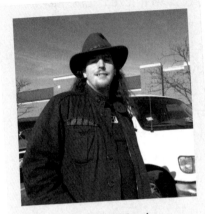

Dave, Walker's brother

But his bedroom was an imperfect retreat, we knew, even with noise-canceling headphones on. Through the thin walls, Dave could hear the frustrated voices of his parents trying to steer Walker one way or another. He could hear Walker's shouting and his parents' shouting in response. He could hear Walker's incessant bouncing on a ball or trampoline, his feet hitting the floor or stairs in a loud, intentional thump that shook the walls. He could hear the endless playing and replaying of Walker's favorite country songs and videotapes.

Possessed of uncanny memory skills, Dave could even recite whole 25-minute Disney stories from heart. Even when his parents were cool and cheerful and handling Walker well, he could feel their tension in his bones and knew that, maybe not in the next few minutes, maybe not this evening even, but sooner or later, Ellen or I would erupt in frustration.

In his room or out of the house, Dave still vibrated with the stress of living with his brother.

So, from his point of view, Walker's new living arrangement was an unmixed blessing. In addition to easing the tension of daily existence, the change meant that Dave could have more attention from his parents, or at least his dad. In the division of labor that was parenthood, I had become Walker's default parent and Ellen had become Dave's. Walker needed active-participant guidance akin to a personal trainer: being with him could be an exhausting physical workout. Restless and kinetic by nature, I slipped easily into this role. Ellen, on the other hand, was a gifted social creature, able to charm doctors, teachers, and therapists in a way I couldn't dream of. She was far more suited than I to the handling of the educational and social and medical issues Dave ended up facing.

His troubles were many: a victim of sudden-onset and severe OCD in the third grade, he spent many months at the National Institutes for Health in Bethesda in a clinical study involving plasmapheresis treatments. Ellen lived with Dave at the NIH for many months, noting with awe how upbeat and stoical Dave was about all the tedious, invasive tests he underwent. The study was based on the theory that OCD could appear suddenly in a child through undetected strep infections. The medical team replaced the blood and thus ridded it of antibodies and—presto!—no more OCD. The therapy worked, at least until the next strep infection. So Dave continued to be plagued with the problem in one way or another for years afterward. His experience was illuminating in important ways. The theory—confirmed by the study—was that misfirings of the autoimmune system could result in antibodies invading the brain. This idea—that OCD and possibly autism itself might be at their roots an autoimmune problem—has been the main model that makes sense to Ellen and me, a model that we think will bear therapeutic fruit someday.

Dave also suffered from Addison's disease—the failure of the adrenal gland to produce cortisone. The extreme rarity of this condition (President John Kennedy was the most famous victim of it) in someone as young as Dave caused Ellen and me and his doctors to miss it for years. His listlessness, his anger, his failure to eat well, the spreading dark patches all over his body—all features of Addison's—were symptoms missed by the doctors at the NIH. At last admitted to the hospital in near-critical condition at age 16, he received the correct diagnosis and medication and he improved in every way. Ellen and I realized with horror that he had stoically suffered with it for years, possibly since age eight.

Guilt, like a relentless zombie in a horror flick, has dogged every step of this parenting journey of ours.

The other burden Dave carried was intellectual giftedness. Of course, this term "gifted" is one of the big eye-rollers in the land of child rearing. Nearly all parents believe their kid is "gifted" in some way. This is a good thing: parents should be child-boosters, not negaters. But "gifted" was a label hung on Dave early on by the Chicago Public Schools, and it was one we clung to with some desperation. Thrown out of four preschools for his impulsive behavior, usually accompanied by some teacher's dire prediction about his coming scholastic career, he scored very high on a test for giftedness, and so we ran with this result.

His impulsiveness could best be seen in a defining habit of his as a three-, four-, and five-year-old. He might be watching TV or looking at a book or talking to us when suddenly, out of the blue, he'd stand up, say "Boop boop boop!" and start to skip around the house telling a story. Not just a "story," however, but a real narrative with carefully chosen words, audible deletions, corrections, and plot lines. People told us, "They're so cute at this age. Treasure these days, for they won't last." But they did last, and continued into young adulthood. At 18, he no longer said "Boop boop boop" and no longer skipped around in a circle, but I liked to think a silent "Boop boop boop" thrummed in his head when he sat down at his computer to write each day.

Dave's label was a blessing of sorts. He became a special ed student, with an aide in the classroom, but in a gifted program. The very first day of elementary school set the pattern for the next 12 years. One of his teachers decided that the first thing the students needed to learn was how horrible they really were, to drive some of that self-esteem-boosting "gifted" stuff out of their systems—never mind that this was a gifted school. She lined them up around the classroom in the first five minutes of class and had them perform this exercise: One by one, turn to the student next to them and say, "I'm very sorry for what I did. Can you forgive me?" (Note: This is in a modern school in the 1990s in the United States of America, not Charles Dickens's hellish Dotheboy's Hall in nineteenth-century Britain.)

When it came to Dave's turn, he knelt down on the floor and looked up into the next girl's eyes and shouted with an Al Jolson-ish swagger, "I'm very sorry I offended ya, Susie! Can ya FORGIVE me?" This marked the beginning of endless trips to the principal's office and endless trips to school for Ellen as she fought battle after battle with the school system to keep Dave enrolled and ensure that he was educated sensitively and intelligently. It was an education in human nature for Ellen: schooling in how to deal with people, how to be supportive of them and yet firm at the same time. She always kept in mind a saying of her mother's: "People will be everything you expect them to be and nothing more." I always summarized her style as "Flatter, flatter, flatter, then hint at possible litigation."

But being gifted was also a barrier. Dave suffered from depression. He had a therapist, Rich Arend, an excellent, intelligent, supportive child psychologist, who attended meetings with Ellen and stood by Dave in his battles with the Chicago Public Schools. He gave Dave advice such as "Don't mock the teacher in class. Save up all your stories for when you get home or see me. Then we can all laugh at the teacher together." Through it all, Dave's own unstoppable creativity saved him. He could come back home feeling sad and eventually we'd hear him laughing in his room over a new story he was writing. Dave was resourceful and resilient. We believed that a quieter home and more normalized lifestyle could only help him.

→ ←

The challenge was for Ellen and Bob to try to lower their pulses, to let the quiet of the half-empty nest seep into their nervous systems and calm them down, now that they were "free" Monday through Friday. So we set about getting some things done. We cleaned the house a bit. We hired repairmen when we could. We went out to a movie or concert once in a while on a Friday night. I graded papers in peace and quiet—or rather, I made a pot of coffee, placed my students' essays on a clipboard, counted them, took out my grade book and blue pen, read the first three, counted how many I had left, then turned on a rerun of *Law and Order: Criminal Intent*. I was beginning to discover that Walker's interruptions were just an excuse; I continued to race through the papers from 9 p.m. to 1 a.m. on Sunday nights. The biggest boon was that Ellen could return to work. She got a job writing grants for a foundation—one that permitted her to work at home—and we started to make inroads on our heavy debts.

Actually relaxing, however, was pretty much beyond us. We did know ourselves to be quite lucky in several respects. The biggest, most fabulous fact was that Walker lived just a 20-minute drive away. Many parents of disabled children would kill to have a CILA so close to the family home. The closest living arrangements many Illinois parents could find were out of state. Seeing their child meant a long drive, even a stay in a motel. But we were close enough to pick him up every Saturday morning and have him home with us for two days out of every week. (This commitment, though, meant we were still unavailable to friends on weekends, making us seem like childcare fanatics.)

So we had both the good fortune and the tension of picking him up every Saturday and devoting the following 48 hours to him. If we saw him only once a month, say, and never brought him home, we would not have been so in touch with how things were going with him. He would have sunk, by default as it were, out of mind a bit. But we were always at least semi-aware of his changing moods, his health, his medications, his activities, his housemates, his diet. We became friendly with the staff and his teachers at the vocational center; they became "favorites" on our cell phones.

We knew, or thought that we knew, how he was doing week by week. Thus we were able to maintain—and neurotically made sure that we did maintain—the level of anxiety that we had become accustomed to.

CHAPTER 5

Friends

ON A COLD, SUNNY spring day, Walker and I were trekking through a North Side neighborhood having a fine time, except for the fact that This Guy was tagging along. Everything was OK, as far as I was concerned, except for the presence of This Guy. He seemed to think the story here was that he and Walker were doing their usual thing, whereas I knew the story was about Walker and me. Hadn't my son and I, for some 20 years, traversed, crisscrossed, explored, even gotten slightly lost covering the vast territory of Chicago north of the Madison Street equator and near the lake? We were Lewis and Clark; This Guy could be—maybe—a helpful scout.

But I knew better. Doug, the director of the CILA, had invited me to come along with him and Walker on one of their daily walks through the neighborhood. Walker had been living at the CILA for several weeks and they had already established a routine. After vocational training was over in the mid-afternoon each day, Walker and Doug walked several miles past the bungalows and apartment buildings and on to the lakefront. He was taking me along, I think, because he wanted to reassure me about how happy Walker was with his new life there, and he also was rightly proud of the bond they had established.

And, as far as I could see, Doug was doing spectacularly, even in some ways better than I normally did. Walker seemed to take direction from him better: "Hey, man. Let's not go that way today. Let's go this way." And Walker cheerfully complied! I usually let Walker push me around. If he wanted a rigidly established route for a few weeks, that was OK with me. I knew that suggestions about new directions might mean public wrangling, pulling, and stern insistence that I wasn't up to. For instance, at the Belmont L (Chicago's signature elevated train), if he wanted to take a very long walk, I let him pull me onto a Brown Line train. My desire for the Red Line and a shorter walk on any given day had nothing to do with it.

"Don't pick that up, Walker," Doug said. "Put that back in the garbage can." And he did put the half-filled cup of Coke back in the garbage can! No resistance, no dispute. With me, even though I felt I was hovering like a hawk, Walker could pick up a discarded cup and take a sip of the remaining beverage before I knew he had faked me out. Doug was quick and wise and had the fresh enthusiasm of a new player in a football game. And he could say things in a quiet, self-assured, but commanding way that I knew I couldn't imitate. Even *I* felt like snapping to attention.

All this was absolutely, jubilantly reassuring—but still a little sad for me. I felt that Walker was slipping away from me slightly. I had the feeling that a mother might have about her toddler ignoring her on entering a park and running over to a new friend for the first time—in my son's 22nd year! Walker, of course, had many friends—mainly family, teachers, therapists—but nobody who did what *I did* with him.

It hit me: growing up is hard for parents as well as kids.

→ ←

A tall, good-looking, amiable man in his late 40s, Doug was exactly the right person to transition a nervous father at a critical moment in the old guy's life as a parent. He paid particular attention to showing me how Walker's world was continuing in familiar ways, but with significant ratcheting up of all the things necessary for a growing young man.

Take the bedroom. Walker had a room to himself, a colossal improvement over his dining-room sleeping arrangements at home. It was a second-floor corner room with views of trees and grass and attractive neighboring homes. His bed was large and cozy and was covered by comforters of various thicknesses according to the season. Not that the seasons mattered much because the house had central air conditioning, an out-of-reach luxury to his parents. His walls had posters of his country music heroes: Clint Black, Alan Jackson, Toby Keith, and Taylor Swift. He had all his favorite CDs and books, videotapes, and a TV. Ellen, Walker, and I all had input into the layout of this room, but Doug was the guiding hand that made sure it all happened.

There were six other residents in the house, each of whom had their own single room. This in itself was sultanic luxury. Most CILAs in Illinois, because of budget restraints, required two residents to each room, and Walker's odd sleeping habits— he frequently woke up in the middle of the night and stayed awake—would have made any roommate's existence intolerable. It was a toss-up as to which resident in his house had the best living quarters: all the rooms were fine in their own ways.

Indeed, the house was just the sort of place I myself dreamed of living in. A big, sturdy, three-floor old frame structure with a porch (and a swing!), a back yard and front yard, a fireplace, big kitchen, basement, and two bathrooms, this was a place built for *living*, for *fun*. The heavy oak woodwork everywhere, the stairs that went up and up, the hidden rooms and closets, the narrow hallways turning every which way—it reminded me pleasantly of sprawling houses I had boarded in as a grad student in Evanston. It also seemed like a fantasy of a cool frat house where young adults could stretch a bit, feel a bit free, feel as if they were doing what people their age do. Walker certainly felt this way. Every Saturday, he eagerly came home with us for his familiar stuff: Zoo–Train–Walk, videos, puzzles, food, reassuring household chatter. But every Sunday evening he just as eagerly ran back into the house to see his friends, to have his newly developing adult existence.

Sitting next to me in the car and smiling at me on the way back to his house on Sunday night, I imagined him saying:

This is great, Dad. This is what I've always wanted. Doug is really cool. My room is great, too. And it's my room! It's not the living room and not a room I have to share with Dave. It's a busy place and I love all the activity in the place. We have a regular routine each day and you know how I like that. At home, I feel like what we're going to do is too much up in the air, too random, if you know what I mean. Here, they're always cheerful, especially Doug. He isn't so afraid of letting me do something new or giving me a job to do. I love jobs, a lot. I love doing laundry and especially vacuuming. I'm not very good at it, but I love to try. And they're always paying attention to me. At home you grade papers and watch TV, Mom cleans and writes, Dave's in his room, and I feel like I'm in the way. Here, everything is geared to me and my housemates. It's better, believe me, Dad. Don't worry so much!

Over the next weeks and months, Doug told me stories about his adventures with Walker that amazed and reassured me, and caused no small amount of envy. He seemed to be doing better with Walker than I did, but how could that be? For example, I claimed credit for teaching Walker to be a smooth supermarket shopper. This was one of my greatest achievements. I deserved, I thought, a trophy of some sort: a tiny gold me pushing a tiny gold cart with a happy, tiny, gold young man beside me. It had taken years, but I finally had reached a point where he was a helpful companion in a store and not a time bomb.

There had been many stages. Between the ages six and 12 or so, he would walk along beside me fine for a while but at some point might take off running, fast, to the opposite end of the store. Or he might start shouting, or lie down flat and refuse to move in the checkout line, or spit (a nearby shopper would get a *Did-I-just-see-that?* look on her face), or tug and push and insist on leaving and force me to abandon a cart full of groceries at the furthest end of the store. In his teen years, there was a stage when I was never sure if he'd actually get out of the car in the parking lot and walk into the store with me. (Was he ashamed to be seen with his dad?) I would park the car strategically to minimize the possibility of his walking across a driving lane. Then I'd lecture sternly before exiting: "OK, Walker, if you don't want to go into the store, that's OK, but you *must* stay in the car. I don't want you walking alone through the parking lot. It's not safe. OK?" He'd reply, "OK, Dad." Then I'd run into the store—literally run—and grab a few things.

Sometimes this would work, other times not so much. I would be throwing items into the cart and hear a distant "Ah, ah, ah!" and I'd know: he'd left the car, had navigated the parking lot safely, thank God, and was now somewhere in the store looking for me. The clerks and store personnel knew us well and were familiar with our routines. We were the nice, zany, but sometimes alarming shopping duo. On occasion it seemed to me that I could see one of our cashier friends quietly reassuring a customer, "No, they aren't really dangerous. They're good."

Controlling Walker was one problem. Controlling my embarrassment was another. It took me years to develop a thick skin about small public humiliations—longer, I think, than it might take other parents. But I gave myself (I was the principal family shopper) enormous credit: my son was not hidden away. He was out in the world, mixing with other citizens of the world, and he clearly loved it. He always had an eager, happy look on his face during our daily or twice-daily outings—walking, going to playgrounds, museums, supermarkets, big-box stores. His world was spacious, sprawling, colorful, and fun. As time went by, he became easier and easier to be out with in public. We still had limits, of course. Sitting through a movie or concert was close to impossible. Long lines were trouble. But he became ever more relaxed and self-assured, and I developed the hide of a rhinoceros.

→ ←

Doug came along at just the right moment. He was able to see much more potential in all this achievement than I did. He refused to push a cart—Walker had to do it. He refused to pay the cashier—Walker had to. He didn't go down the aisle and buy Tide—Walker had to manage it. This ability to push and teach, inspire and make novel demands was exhilarating. Finally, more was being expected of Walker and he was proud to perform. He felt the confidence Doug had in him, and this emboldened him to try new things. Once they were in a 7-11 store and Doug noticed that Walker was glancing at the *Sports Illustrated* swimsuit issue. "You like that, Walker? Why don't you buy it?" So Walker took out *his own* wallet and paid for it with *his own* cash from a small allowance he got weekly.

They were in a shoe store trying on shoes, but had no luck. So, on leaving, Doug said, "Put your shoes back on, Walker." He pulled on one shoe and then quickly pulled it off. "Come on, now. Put on your shoe, Walker." He tried again and then jerked it off.

"Barrassed," Walker said.

"What do you mean? Come on, you can do it."

"Barrassed," he said again.

Doug took a look at the shoe, peered inside, and spotted the problem: Walker's sock was tucked into the toe and so he couldn't pull the shoe all the way on. The wonderful thing, of course, was the exchange—Walker using a word for the first time and at the right time and actually mentioning a *feeling* he had. This was brand-new stuff. Ellen and I were thrilled to hear about it, but in truth I felt a little "barrassed" myself. I was great at getting Walker outdoors but poor at inching him to responsible, competent, and confident action. Doug was skilled at this—ushering him into a brave new world.

→ ←

Doug, as head of the CILA, set the tone for the place and every staff member. He often spoke of his job as a late-found calling in life—a vocation. He felt paternal toward the residents, all of whom were in their twenties. He loved and befriended Walker and his housemates, and they felt they were special to him. The staff, as often happens at a workplace, shared the attitude of the boss: an intelligent, empathetic, gentle, fun ethos pervaded the place. This was quite remarkable. The pay was low and for nearly all workers was considered an interim job—to help pay for school, to survive in a gap between this and more permanent work. Much was demanded of them for a position that gave no payoff in social status or monthly check. The real rewards of the job were intangible and possible only to those with big hearts: a sense of pride in helping others and the friendships forged by those with a gift for making connections with low-functioning autistic people.

A parent could truly understand how arduous this job really was. Throughout his life Walker constantly presented Ellen and me with issues that made us feel completely out of our depth. I had a Ph.D. and taught college classes but still, even with my awesome high-wattage brain, I knew that teaching was a visit to a beach in Maui compared with the problems Walker presented daily. I often left for work with the guilty-but-not-all-that-guilty feeling that somebody else (now, who would that be?) would have to handle things. After all, I was *the breadwinner*.

My work as a teacher was satisfying. I had a decent income, a sense of career advancement, and a certain status in the community. To be sure, I wasn't Kim Kardashian or Donald Trump, but I could hold my head reasonably high. I taught Freshman Composition to mainly English-as-a-second-language students, and therefore knew that I was doing something valuable. I was providing them with a skill they would definitely need in their new lives in America. They were grateful to me and often told me so. By and large, I worked hard. I excavated whatever reserves of skill I had to handle my classes in creative or novel ways. But if they couldn't learn the material, well, they failed and had to take the class again. I didn't have to keep seeing them every day, day in, day out, night in, night out, and be confronted with my own failure to get the message across. It would be frustrating, true, when some repeated direction would be ignored, or if I hadn't done an adequate job of explaining something, but, hey, it was their funeral, so to speak. And I had the evidence of much success: the vast majority of them learned the material and passed. I was a "good teacher" and knew it.

Things are not so cut and dried for an aide working in a group home. She might try to teach a resident to wash his hands and approach the task in a variety of creative ways. But no matter how creative and no matter how many times she tries, the resident may not ever actually do it. Ever. But her job is to keep trying and not stop trying. Each night, after not washing his hands, the resident might not brush his teeth without heavy direction and then might not take off his shirt, not put it in the laundry, and then not put on his pajamas, despite many many hopeful, enthusiastic, cheerful, agonizing, dogged, loving, maddening instructions from the aide. When something surprising happens—say, he begins to wash his hands without prompting—he might not follow through and finish. And then the next night he may forget he ever made progress the previous night. But the aide can't give him an F and he doesn't thank her for trying. She can't think, "Well, it's his funeral," and smugly remind herself of her many other successes. She simply moves on to another resident and yet another with similar issues. She can feel like Sisyphus, meaninglessly pushing a rock, or rather three or four rocks, up a mountain only to watch them all roll down again.

This kind of work, in a fair world, would be rewarded with spectacular salaries and great prestige. The inner reserves of talent, character, intelligence, patience, wisdom, and empathy required to do this job, and do it well, are vast. On the other hand, it's very hard to imagine a hedge fund Master of the Universe staying focused, with kindliness, on the failed hand-washer. But, as most of us learn by age ten, it's not a fair world or even nearly fair: "The race is not to the swift, nor the battle to the strong, neither yet bread to the wise, nor yet riches to men of understanding…" etc., etc.

→ ←

Doug was one kind of friend and role model for Walker: the calm, deliberate, and mature adult man. Nic was another kind of friend and role model: the kind, fun, and free-wheeling rock star. A few years after the opening of the CILA, Nic was hired as a staff member and had a special assignment to focus on Walker. He turned out to be the fantasy friend of a twenty-something young man. Not much older than Walker, Nic was tall and dashingly handsome, with a leading man's profile, long black hair, and Johnny Depp feel for couture: one day he'd wear a tight black cowboy shirt, shorts, and hipster black silver-studded boots; the next day he'd appear in corduroy slacks, red scarf, and black t-shirt.

Relaxed and confident, he was up for anything, any time of day. Walker liked country music? They went to a country music bar. Walker liked getting around the city? They rode the buses and trains everywhere, into every sort of neighborhood. Walker liked big outdoor Chicago events? Out they went to

Occupy Chicago and did this, as a rock star might say, with a bullet.

It was the fall of 2011 when the Occupy movement was in full swing. Young adults especially were marching, sitting in, and protesting in the name of the 99 percent against the greed and corruption of the 1 percent. Their motto: "We kick the ass of the ruling class." It was a movement uncannily similar to the student protests of the Vietnam era when I was in college, and I admit my own baby-boomer nostalgia neurons were jumping. Nic thought it was just the thing for friends like Walker and him to join, but not—heaven forbid—in any predictably dull way. It was a moment, like every Nic moment, for the panache of a personal statement. It was a serious street protest for sure, but it was also clearly a moment for street theater, for performance art.

He and Walker went out to vintage clothing shops and put together cheap black tuxedos for the occasion. What better irony than men who look vaguely Wall Street tycoon-ish marching in an anti-Wall Street parade? And what better irony than to baffle the bourgeois marchers themselves with a little show within the show? It was so very Nic and so very exciting for Walker. To be with his friend, to be out with the crowd, to be in the center of his city's action: a dream afternoon.

When they arrived downtown where the crowd was gathering, several people urged them to move to the front of the march. They looked good, and if one didn't look too closely, ultra-respectable. It was tempting. But although Nic was a showman, he was there for a more serious reason than street theater: to give his friend a slice of the real life he craved. Walker was grinning and game for anything, to be sure, but Nic knew that at any moment Walker's nerve could crack and he'd have to light out for the territory, to head out on his own route away from the overstimulation of thousands of shouting people. It was always like this with Walker and crowds. Yes, he wanted to be there at the center of the action: to be at the Chicago Marathon, to be at the St. Patrick's Day Parade, to be at the breast cancer run, but only for a while and only if he knew he could punt when the pressure got to be too much. If a camera had followed them, an Occupy Chicago TV news story could have turned into the autism viral video of the week. So they marched along in the middle of the crowd and elected to exit 25 minutes later.

Another Nic-inspired street theater moment turned out even better. The following spring, during the NATO summit meeting in Chicago, of course Nic had to be where the action was: in the middle of the spectacular, cast-of-thousands street protest. Out they went again, this time with no special costumes and *no backpacks, please!* They tagged along with the crowd for a while and Walker was enjoying the show until he hit his tipping point and had to bolt. But they were now trapped in a sea of shouting people with no escape in sight. So Nic pulled Walker through the crowd until he found a police officer and told her something like "This is more than a NATO protest, officer— this is autism!" She sized up the situation instantly and escorted them to one of many idling buses, presumably waiting to escort crowds of protesters to jail just in case there was a repeat of the 1968 Democratic Convention incident—one I remembered well—involving police and anti-war demonstrators. (Ah, be still, my baby-boomer nostalgic heart.)

It was one of the monster articulated buses, a kind of double-bus, a vehicular parade all by itself. Nic and Walker got on and sat near the front. They were the only passengers. "Where do you guys want to go?" the driver said.

"Well, actually we're not close—up on the far North Side," Nic explained.

"Good," the driver said. He closed the door and off the three of them went, Nic thinking, *What the…?* and Walker grinning and staring ahead and probably thinking, *Of course this is happening! I'm with Nic!*

→ ←

Ellen and I knew Nic to be a cool friend and guide for Walker, but we had no idea just how cool he was exactly. In short, tentative conversations we discovered he'd graduated from Ohio University, Ellen's alma mater, and he mentioned that he and his friends had done some comedy sketches and posted them on YouTube. We didn't think much more about it than *How nice that Nic dreams of a more glamorous life and career.* One day he let us know that he and his friends were doing a show of comic sketches at the Music Box Theater and maybe we'd like to go. We thought, *Huh? That's a very large venue. What does he plan to do there?*

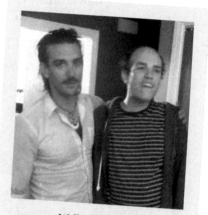

Walker and Nic

Dave and I thought we'd drop by and check it out. When we got there, we discovered there was no "dropping by." There was a line over a block long just to get into the theater. Chatting with the people around us, we discovered that Nic's troupe—he was the leader—had a devoted cult following. Called Everything is Terrible, the players had a *Saturday Night Live* vibe, but their bits were edgier, wackier, more *out there*. The large theater was crowded and Nic was clearly the star. The audience was convulsed with laughter and obviously familiar with the group and, in the manner of Monty Python devotees, thrilled to be seeing them live. Soon afterward Nic took a leave of absence from the CILA and went on tour with Everything, filling venues in 50 places all over the country.

So much for the just-above-minimum-wage staffer at a group home and so much for the preconceptions of 60-something parents. The lesson we repeated incessantly to people—*Never underestimate Walker*—was one we had to keep learning about everybody else in our lives.

→ ←

The move to the group home, so frightening to Ellen and me, was becoming one of the best things that ever happened to Walker. He was getting his wish, getting out in the world and living in his own house—in his own cool frat house actually—and feeling the excitement of young adulthood.

And, for a while, his world just kept getting better.

CHAPTER 6

"I Work There"

"WALKER DOESN'T POINT."

This was a phrase that seemed to sum up Walker's entire problem for us. In talking to new evaluators and therapists and teachers and doctors, "Walker doesn't point" was the first volley in our unvarying speech explaining the depth of his difficulty. Telling a school evaluator "He's autistic" was a non-starter. Every single person's—indeed, every single expert's—definition of autism was unpredictable. The word "autistic" was vague and elastic, conveying different things to different people. But not pointing, like not nodding yes and no, is a vivid disability that nails the issue. It was the starting point of his trouble.

He pointed plenty before age three. He'd read books aloud with his finger following the words; he'd pointed and counted plastic animal figures he'd line up in a row. But that ended when his silence began at three, the traditional start of autism for many children. We would beg him to point to the toy he wanted, to the color red in a book, to the picture of a horse, to the moon. These were all things we knew he could do because he had done them, yet he wouldn't. He seemed to be saying, *Look. You're not roping me into this conversation. I know I can't talk. I feel in over my head here. I don't like how my voice sounds. In fact, I'm just too distracted all the time to follow this conversational avenue you want to go down. So please stop.*

When he did talk, mainly repeating words we'd asked him to say or giving one-word answers to questions, he'd tag a "t" sound to the end of the word as though to make it *his* word, not ours. "Chair" became "chair-t," "apple" became "apple-t," and "cookie" became "cookie-t." (*I'll cave and say a few words, guys. But I'll say them* my *way.*) Not pointing was a piece of this. If he pointed, he knew that wouldn't be the end of it. Mom and Dad would expect more, and more was exactly what he didn't want. To me, his not pointing was also an aspect of what I can only call his "physical shyness." Hammering a nail was out of the question: he would/could never wield a hammer hard enough. Washing himself was always an issue because he wouldn't/couldn't put in the effort to scrub. Hugging someone was a problem, not because he was averse to contact (far from it), but because he wouldn't/couldn't apply the slight pressure of his hand. His autism sometimes seemed to be shyness pushed to its ultimate extreme.

So one day when the three of us were in the car driving near the vocational center and he actually pointed at the building and audibly said, "I work there," we were dumbstruck. (Admittedly, we were dumbstruck for only about five seconds because Ellen and I never stop talking, but we did pause noticeably.) "Yes, Walker. That's where you work! What do you do there, man?" I said, excited and pushing him, hoping to lure him, trick him, entice him into dialogue. No answer.

Ellen pressed. "This is where you do your work. You have friends here. What's your favorite thing to do at voc? Do you have fun? Do you like setting tables?" No answer. But he had said it—a real English sentence; our ears had not deceived us.

And he had pointed! We took it as proof that he was proud of what he was doing there—proud enough to break his vow of silence and endure the unwelcome onslaught of questions from Mom and Dad. Throughout his life, at random-seeming moments, Walker had made comments that took our breath away. These rare comments were casual, offhand, flip—*What do you mean? I talk. Of course I do.* The words always begged the question: If he can make any comment at all, if the potential is clearly there, why can't he do it more often? What exactly is happening in his brain? Why does the verbal component switch on only briefly, maddeningly?

But "I work there" plus pointing was not merely random; it arose from excitement and pride in his new life. Having a job was a huge fact worth communicating about.

→ ←

Any brief spark of speech, any new curious movement of the head, any small sudden interest in something that we had never witnessed before was a this-just-into-the-newsroom event to Ellen and me. Was Walker suddenly starting to gaze at the side-view mirror out the car window? Ellen and I saw this as suggesting a multitude of interior mental worlds. Is he safety conscious? Is he mimicking his dad driving the car and feeling responsible somehow? Does he dream of driving himself, like any 22-year-old, and imagine what choices he'd make about changing lanes? Could he, in fact, safely drive the car if given the chance? (He won't get the chance.)

This excited speculation may seem weird in itself. Walker was now 22 and the conventional wisdom was that autism was a static, permanent condition. When he was three years old, a pediatric neurologist pronounced his doom: "I hold out no hope for this child." In the language of the 1980s autism world, we were supposed to do our "grieving" and get on with life. With luck, Walker could learn certain life skills such as bathing and cleaning and brushing his teeth, but he should be—in the kindest possible way and in the best possible meaning of the word and with all the loving care in the world—written off. The message was clear: autistic people were all the same and fundamentally uninteresting. We rejected this idea strongly. We knew our boy as intelligent, capable of great change, and riddled with supposedly non-autistic personality traits. We loved him, we liked him, we thought him fascinating as hell. So-called "denial" became our proud mission in life.

The infuriating word to us was the third person plural pronoun, "they," referring to people with autism. It was a trigger word that brought out the worst in us. We'd be speaking to a caregiver or doctor or teacher and discussing Walker's motivation for something he did. Suddenly, the word would appear, as in "Well, Mr. and Mrs. Hughes, that's just something *they* do." The word "just" was often part of the sentence, for the meaning was clear: Stop looking for motives. Stop trying to imagine what Walker's up to. He's *autistic*, get it? He's not interesting, like you or me or the next-door neighbor. He's part of a category and that's where the discussion ends. The word would bring out our curious marital dynamic. Ellen would listen politely, perhaps roll her eyes, and patiently try to get back to why-Walker-Hughes-did-something. I would stand there, looking dark and angry, hoping the steam I felt coming out of my ears wasn't visible, and, on a good day, actually keep my mouth shut. On the way home, Ellen would have to endure my explosions of helpless post-facto angry put-downs. Then she would have to remind me, "There's no sense in yelling at people. Besides, you never know when you might need them later."

We knew that the they-sayers had a dumb and obvious point. Viewed from a distance, Walker was "just like" his autistic classmates. He couldn't converse and, true to predictions from his childhood, had made no dramatic progress in speech over many years of training. He couldn't take complicated directions and do a job and keep at it for hours. He couldn't play a competitive game competitively. A list of his shortcomings in daily competence could go on and on and look similar to that of his low-functioning autistic peers. But this distant view shut down understanding. It relied on a label, as though naming in and of itself explained something; as though an astronomer, with a patronizing smile, had said to a mystified stargazer, "Oh, that's just what we experts call an Unidentified Flying Object." And it left out the fascinating, troubling, mysteriously happy Walker Hughes who ached to communicate every moment of his life. A caregiver who thought of Walker first and foremost (and sometimes last) as "an autistic" was no friend at all, just a tauntingly close emblem of a friend, a loneliness-generator.

⇀ ↽

Walker had, at various times, three jobs at voc. One was setting tables at a nursing home and emptying trash. Another was cleaning up at a popular restaurant in the Loop. And another was delivering college newspapers at various points on a North Side college campus. Each job lasted only one or two hours of the work day. At each one he had a "coach" who accompanied him, coaxed him, guided him every step of the way. It wasn't "working" in the sense of a person actually slogging through an eight-hour day in a fast-food restaurant; it was more like an introduction to work, a representation of work. Getting Walker, or any of the clients at voc, to stay on a task doing something independently for eight hours every day—the dream!—was effectively impossible. But the small amount of work he did do made a very big difference in his life. He was enthusiastic, proud, engaged. It was part of a new adult identity for him.

The head of the vocational training program and Walker's dear friend at voc was Daryl (not his real name). He had worked with Walker for years as a teacher in Walker's special school and so knew him well. Having Daryl at a job site with him was a confidence builder for Walker. Daryl was friendly, handsome, kind, soft-spoken, and, it seemed to us, had a natural talent for helping autistic people, for treating them as friends and not victims with labels. He had a hard task. I had a pretty good idea what Daryl faced as his job coach. As Walker's valet—his Jeeves—I knew exactly how difficult it was to get Walker to do something and keep him at it. So I was delighted every day to know that Walker had Daryl, a familiar face, a friend at his side every day to guide him.

The rest of the staff at voc was equally gifted. Usually college students working part-time, they approached their jobs with smiles, enthusiasm, and realistic expectations. In the early days at voc, the staff seemed to approach their low-paid work with something like religious zeal. It was clearly more than a job to them; it was a vocation. In addition to Daryl, Walker had several job coaches, each of whom treated Walker as a friend.

Of lesser value, but still important, was what Walker did the rest of the day at voc. The center was basically a big room with tables. The job of the staff was to keep about 20 clients (the number grew year by year) busy learning skills. They worked on computers, they worked on reading and writing, they played games. But the staff was up against some immovable obstacles. One was the functioning level of the clients themselves. The goal of the center was to take some of the lowest-functioning autistic people and give them work in the community. This was quixotic: some of the clients couldn't even go out in a van and do something as engaged with normal living as emptying trash or setting a table. There were no "high-functioning" young people there who could converse and learn a complex job.

Another problem—the biggest problem—was money. It takes plenty of financing to pay staff and make connections with businesses and write grant proposals to get money from government and foundations. The center was partially funded by the state, but Illinois was famous for its scandalously weak support for adults with disabilities. Fundraising was therefore very important, especially for a group home and vocational center that were quite small and not connected to a larger agency of some kind. Ellen for a time worked as a writer for the center and won grants from organizations such as Autism Speaks and other more local funders, and she was instrumental in helping to establish both the group home and the vocational center. But money for grant writers was itself a luxury for an organization struggling just to breathe from day to day.

Voc wasn't ideal. It was noisy and chaotic. Any time Ellen and I stopped by, the staff was friendly and upbeat, but many clients seemed to be doing nothing at all. As time went by and more clients arrived, this problem of noise and crowding only became worse. The burgeoning population at the center was no surprise to us. We knew autism rates in the country were exploding and saw Walker's immediate world as a microcosm of the problem. In 1988, when he was about two and half, an acquaintance suggested that he could be autistic. We mentioned this to Ann Jernberg, a distinguished and brilliant child psychologist friend of ours, who said, "Walker's autistic? Your loving little boy? No way." She added, "Autism is very rare. There can't be more than two autistic children in the whole Chicago area."

Ann was in the mainstream of thinking about autism back then. The mere fact that a statistic didn't spring to her lips at the time was an indicator of how far below the medical radar autism was flying in the 80s. According to the Environmental Protection Agency, the trend upwards in the number of autistic children ballooned sometime between 1988 and 1992 from 6 in 10,000 to 24 in 10,000.[1] Every few years in Walker's life we saw the number climb from 1 in 166 births to 1 in 150 to the current 1 in 68. However the numbers were arrived at and despite criticism of the assumptions behind the diagnoses, there was no doubt that something very, very serious was happening, something of critical concern medically and politically and socially. Walker was part of the vanguard of a stark increase in numbers, and his peers from the 1980s were starting to become adults.

Evidence of the growth in numbers hit us in casual conversation constantly through the years. In the early days when we mentioned Walker's autism, we had to launch into our layman's lecture about what the word meant. As time went by, the word was on more and more lips until any mention that our son was autistic brought out sometimes tentative, sometimes eager statements about the son, the niece, the granddaughter, the boss's ten-year-old who had been diagnosed and a

---

1   McDonald, M.E. and Paul, J.F. (2010) "Timing of Increased Autistic Disorder Cumulative Incidence." *Environmental Science and Technology* 44, 6, 2112–2118.

description of the anxiety that was churning in the family. This explosion in autism diagnoses was surely, in part, a result of a growing clinical separation between the categories "retarded" and "autistic," especially since many autistic people could score well on IQ tests. But it was also quite real. These parents knew they weren't being tricked into some fad diagnosis; they knew their kid was in huge trouble. The bottom line was "Can I imagine my child supporting herself independently and living safely when I'm gone?" For a growing number the answer was no.

So whenever we stepped into the voc center's noisy but friendly world, we knew we were looking at Walker's generation: the children of baby boomers and beyond, a new population with a problem only dimly addressed by government.

→ ←

Whenever we looked at the big picture—Walker's future and prospects for a happy life—Ellen and I had reasons for high anxiety. Would the program last despite its financial shakiness? Would Walker continue to thrive in the face of inevitable changes in his living arrangements and his work? Would he always be surrounded by good people who tried, as his earnest staff was trying, to see the world through his eyes?

But Ellen and I were old hands at staying focused on the small picture—the smaller the better. In *The Right Stuff*, Tom Wolfe describes how, when a plane was going down, test pilots wouldn't freeze or panic but rather keep steely focus on the nitty-gritty question: "OK. What do I do next?" This was our goal: to be brave parents with the right stuff, to keep our eyes about one to 24 hours ahead, and avoid screaming, "Oh my God" as the plane went down.

And by and large, overall, in the main, and much of the time, we did exactly that.

→ ←

Walker was currently thriving, so we were thriving too. We were enthusiastic boosters. In one grant proposal after another, Ellen referred to the group home and voc center as a "model program." It certainly was a model program for the Hugheses.

As the next few years went by, Walker was even showing resilience in the face of changes. The staff was always in flux. Job coaches and aides at the group home would leave abruptly for "real" jobs. Doug, the dedicated head of the CILA and Walker's dear friend, was promoted to a job overseeing several group homes and was replaced by Caroline, a special education major who was aiming for graduate work. Instead of this being a problem, however, the transition for Walker was seamless. Caroline quickly became another good friend.

In fact, in the over-fond minds of Walker's parents, Caroline was even the *girl*friend Walker never had. She took him on little date-like excursions to the Loop and around the city, if one's idea of a date is going to a downtown McDonalds on the L, walking into a couple of stores, and riding back on the L. Once, sitting on the Red Line train and rattling north, Walker turned to her, smiled, and said, "Thanks."

"What did you say, Walker?" Caroline asked, amazed. A few minutes passed.

He turned and whispered, "I had a good time." I'm sure Caroline did her best to ratchet up this moment into something more with questions and comments about the day they'd just shared or what they were about to do—everybody who knows him dreams of Walker breaking through and speaking his mind. But, of course, no more follow-up miracles ensued.

When Caroline reported this splash of dialogue to Ellen and me, we levitated for a couple of days. Caroline was our living doll, our darling daughter-in-law, our friend. In the coming years she would go out to eat with us and became a source of ideas about how to help Walker and encourage him to bloom. In fact, Nic and Caroline became good friends with each other, almost like stand-in parents for Walker, and his actual parents started to really relax—almost too much so.

Caroline, like Nic and Doug, treated Walker like that stunning phenomenon: a normal person. They watched him for all the signs of who he was and what he was thinking and tried to infer his tastes, his wishes, his dreams. They peered or attempted to peer through autism's thick screen to detect the person on the other side.

They had the wisdom to beware of the Unintended Outcome of the Negative Self-Fulfilling Prophecy.

Negative Self-Fulfilling Prophecy: Based on previous experience taking him downtown, the aide predicts that when she takes Walker to the St. Patrick's Day Parade he will show no interest. He will ignore the parade and tug her away from it to go in his own direction. She bases this prediction also on what she has read about autistics: *they* hate noise, *they* hate crowds, *they* are object-oriented and not people-oriented.

Natural Consequence of Negative Self-Fulfilling Prophecy: Despite the sad prediction, the aide decides to valiantly attempt the expedition. They do go downtown and, sure enough, Walker does shun the parade. In fact, at the very moment when the aide and Walker emerge from the subway to see the parade in progress, Walker quickly scoots in another direction. The aide feels what a waste of time the outing has been. But she is consoled by one thing: the Prophecy was accurate!

Unintended Outcome of Negative Self-Fulfilling Prophecy: The aide never tries such an outing again and spreads the word to other staff members: Walker hates parades. Outcome: As a result, another sliver of light and life slips behind the cataracts that creep along Walker's field of vision of what's possible for him in the world.

Nic and Caroline and Doug avoided this scenario by being humbler about what was really going on, by acknowledging how much they didn't know about what was happening in his head. They tried not to assume, to predict. They just kept their eyes open to the moment. And they knew: life can surprise you. They watched Walker carefully. Did he look at the parade at all? How did he respond, even momentarily? What was passing him when he scooted off in another direction? They watched themselves carefully: *How am I behaving? Am I giving off any negative signs, any whiff of hopelessness about the expedition? What have I been saying about the trip? After all, he willingly came along. Have I discouraged him in some way?* They admitted: *I don't know what's really going on in his head. Therefore, I will assume he likes spectacle just as most "normals" do. His avoidance of the show might very well mean that he's overly thrilled. Well, perhaps he can learn to control the thrill just as we all do. We'll try this again.*

As time went by, Ellen and I fell into a comfortable if borderline complacent routine. We picked him up every Saturday morning and kept him with us all day, through the night, and brought him back Sunday evening. Each Sunday when he walked in the door, he would dash in and get a puzzle out of a cabinet, bring it over to the dining-room table, and empty the box in front of him. Then Anastasia, a staff member, would sit with him and be a one-woman cheering section for him as he did the puzzle. As a toddler, he had been a big puzzle fan, even rather precocious and proud of his skill, but as he got older, his interest and ability faded.

Or, rather, this is what we told ourselves. In truth, Ellen and I had ourselves fallen victim to the Unintended Outcome of the Negative Self-Fulfilling Prophecy: we did puzzles with him until he wouldn't do them anymore. Then we, not he, avoided them for years. Anastasia herself had recreated this interest in puzzles, which, of course, was to him a friendship activity. A common stereotype is the solitary autistic person at a table obsessively engaged in an activity: putting Legos together and taking them apart, tearing paper into shreds, playing repetitively with balls or blocks, drawing or coloring. It's a picture of a self-ostracized person, insistently alone. But for Walker the puzzle was more of an excuse for being close to and being busy with a friend. And it didn't hurt that the friend was a tall, model-thin young woman with long hair and a smile on her face.

Anastasia was, in effect, *the* activity.

→ ←

Once when Walker was about five and very beleaguered—his autism was quite apparent and he obviously was well behind his peers in development—a friend gave Ellen and me a compliment that has always stuck: "You guys are doing something right. He's one of the happiest kids I've ever seen." We knew we hadn't created his happiness—it seemed to be built into his DNA. The baby standing in his crib beaming at us in the morning, the toddler in the stroller shouting merrily through the city, the eight-year-old jumping on his trampoline—these exuberant boys seemed to have appeared fully formed. But we did know that the smile could fade and that we could blow it. So this became our goal: to keep the smile on his face. We knew we could worry and worry about his development, feel miserable and anguished about his chances in life, or we could enjoy him, laugh with him, and do what we could to see the possibilities for him.

Four years into his program at the CILA and the voc center, he still had that smile and we still felt triumphant. We had

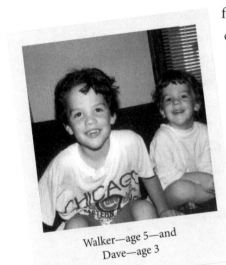

Walker—age 5—and
Dave—age 3

found—indeed, we had helped to create—a fine program for him and a fine house. He was spending his days with people who befriended him and believed in him. We bragged to anyone who would listen about how proud we were of his living situation. When an attorney who knew the autism world well told us that "the best group home you can hope for would rate a B minus," we thought, smugly enough, *Well, Walker's home is a solid A.*

⇢ ⇠

But…but…cracks began appearing in this happy picture.

One Sunday afternoon we took Walker back to his house, and he went to a cabinet to get out a puzzle. He took it to the dining-room table, dumped out its contents, and looked around. Anastasia was nearby, but she was occupied with a new resident of the house, a young man who looked very angry. She was sitting on the couch with him and holding him, actually holding him *down*. We wondered, *What would happen if she let him go?*

I sat with Walker and we did the puzzle together for a while, but after a half hour or so of Ellen trying to make awkward conversation with the critically occupied Anastasia, we decided to leave. As we got into the car, we had our first little chill of guilt about leaving Walker. We were going home to have a pleasant English teacher's Sunday evening of dinner and taking in the current costume drama on PBS. What kind of an evening was Walker going to have? What were we leaving him to? What was going to happen in the next half hour, hour, two hours? What was he thinking?

Gee, thanks, Mom and Dad. You leave me here with nothing to do and nobody to hang out with. And what's with Anastasia? I thought we had a system. I come back and we do a puzzle. She's my good friend and I look forward to doing puzzles with her. She's lots of fun to be with. I'd like to tell her how mad I am or just ask her why she's ignoring me, but I can't. I guess I'll go up to my room and watch the same old videos, but I'm confused and frustrated. The other guys in the house stay in their rooms all the time and the Sunday staff doesn't talk to me unless there's a problem. And who is this new guy? Anastasia isn't doing anything, really. She's just sitting next to him looking like she's ready for trouble. He looks pretty angry.

CHAPTER 7

Fence Me In

MY *LES MISÉRABLES*-STYLE BARRICADE was beautiful, I thought. Atop two dining-room chairs sat the L.L. Bean rocker, upside down, its curved runners sending off a baffling and intimidating message to the invader: *What's this? Surely, this military strategist means business. No one could pass this barrier without heavy equipment.* Next to this was a coffee table with two stools, one sideways, one upended, artfully wedged in a tight formation. Surely the enemy would balk at the stunning, unexpected, and creative immovability of this arrangement. The rough semicircular fence ended at the dining-room table itself, a floor lamp leaning against it at a 45-degree angle, two file boxes weighted with dumb-bells lined up underneath it in case there were any plans to go low and surprise me that way.

I sat behind the barricade in an armchair at 2:30 on a Sunday morning, a flashlight on my lap, layers of blankets over my legs, the perfect picture of a lunatic, but feeling quite pleased with myself. My fort, I knew, was in the optimum strategic spot: the entrance of our narrow hallway at the bottom of the stairs leading up to the bedroom. From here I could block any enemy advance and still visually take in the entire living room. Nothing was going to surprise *me*. The room was dark, but the shadow of the enemy—a tall human form—could be clearly seen against the outdoor light coming faintly through the window blinds.

"Just lie down, Walker. Close your eyes and go to sleep," I said, calmly and gently this time. "We'll have lots of fun tomorrow, but only if you get some sleep tonight."

Without uttering a sound, like a ghost only dimly seen, the form took just three steps back but did not lie down on its bed, the sofa. Instead, it paused only to resume inching steadily forward after a decent interval had passed. This forward movement of the creature, as in a nightmare, was very slow, almost imperceptible. But if I dozed off and stirred awake again, the specter would be at the barricade itself, three feet away from me, looking for the main chance.

I'd become the family's modern major general—off in the silly, mad world of my very tired brain.

→ ←

It had been what was becoming of late a "typical" Saturday night. Earlier, about ten o'clock, Walker announced "Bed into a couch!" This was Walker speak for the opposite: turning our couch into his bed for the night. We had tried several different sleeping arrangements for his one night home per week: a day bed made up for him in our back room, a full-size foam mattress on the floor, even his preferred sleeping spot from his childhood days—the dining-room table moved out, a sleeping bag and mattress where the table had been. But he definitely preferred this arrangement and for a few years had slept peacefully through the night this way.

Lately, though, he had started waking up after sleeping for a couple of hours and staying awake. He'd go to the bathroom and brush his teeth. Then he'd come upstairs to our bedroom, loudly stomping on each carpet-free step, and stand near the bed. We would try to ignore him, hoping he'd just go downstairs again, but this was a pipe dream. He'd tap Ellen on the arm, and do it again until we acknowledged him. It seemed that he wanted the next day to begin, for everybody to get up, turn on the lights, and spin the Earth a little faster so that the next day, and the next, would go by more quickly. It seemed that he wished he had a stationary vehicle like the one in the old movie *The Time Machine*, with a huge spinning wheel and a counter that spun the calendar days ahead in a blur of speed. But to what end? Where did he think this life on fast forward would lead? This question was not an issue to him. It would be enough that we all raced on and on.

→ ←

It was a fatal restlessness, something dismally familiar to us from his childhood but only now making a reappearance. We knew, of course, that he could be having night-time seizures again, as he did as a toddler, but we had been round and round with neurologists over the years in a frustrating attempt actually to determine this medically. We also sensed that his restlessness was a sign of unhappiness: unable to talk about his thoughts and feelings and desires, he tried to control his life circumstances in the only way he thought he could. *OK, I can't determine anything on the index-card list of activities people make for me each day. But maybe, at least, I can accelerate the scenario.*

All this empathetic speculation about his motives would come the next day. In the middle of the night, however, we just wanted to sleep. I was tired from the long fast hike we had made during the day, and I had student essays—lots of them—to grade on Sunday. Then would begin a grim unvarying sequence: We beg him to go back downstairs. He complies and actually gets back to bed. He comes upstairs again, tapping Ellen. I emit varying responses ranging from patience to marginally controlled rage.

My barricade idea was new and had worked for a couple of weeks. Walker was discouraged enough by my fort to go back to sleep. But the idea was controversial. It seemed to Ellen unhinged, but she knew it made her husband feel empowered. To me it was, well, clever, even MacGyver-esque.

→ ←

This night my vigilance wavered. Walker was insistent on his slow zombie walk, his entertaining game with his dad, and I was very sleepy. I must have dozed off for a few minutes because he was suddenly standing right on the other side of the makeshift wall. Then he proceeded to pick up the lamp, slide a box to the side, walk over to me, and tap me on the foot, as if to say, *Let's make breakfast, Dad!* The total ease with which he went through my wall—the *Star Trek* crew transporting themselves at will comes to mind—took my breath away. And my mind.

So Ellen came downstairs to man the battle station while I went upstairs to bed. Under Ellen's watch he fell asleep almost instantly. And I was left to lie awake and ask myself the question that throbbed in my head: *Why?* We had thought, or perhaps just wished very strongly, that he had "grown out" of the small night-time seizures that seemed to plague him when he was very young. Before age 11, he seemed to never get a deep, lengthy night's sleep. The pursuit of confirming the sleep seizures never seemed to end. Thus that newborn baby era of parents getting up at random moments in the night hadn't faded away for years. The only abatement came when a neurologist, Dr. Michael Chez, changed Walker's anti-seizure medication on the educated guess that the night seizures really were occurring. My memory of the bad old days, teaching class, grading papers, and going to department meetings on very little sleep, was still strong. And now those days had returned, although in a minor key. Instead of being a several-times-a-week issue, now it was only Saturday night. But the new wakeful pattern was taking a toll.

Even given that he was having seizures, again: *Why now?* Seizures can be triggered by severe panic or anxiety. Was there some reason he was upset? Was something happening at his group home or vocational center that we didn't know about? We stepped into his group home only twice every weekend, and we knew this was a pretty poor sampling of the stress level in the house. Yet even this limited exposure hinted at something: Anastasia seemed to be a full-time aide to the new very angry-looking client. And there were two other new residents, a young woman and another young man, both of whom looked difficult to live with.

Over the past weeks, we had noticed troublesome things about these new housemates. Tracey (I've changed the names of all Walker's housemates) was a person in constant motion. We rarely saw her actually seated. She seemed to move like a pinball, lurching from dining room to living room to hallway to game room to bathroom in a continuous random trajectory. She often had a small stick in her hand, usually picked up outdoors in the yard, and would suddenly race up to Ellen or me, waving the stick toward our faces. I knew what this was all about and sympathized. She had no parents to come and visit her. She wanted our attention and, unable to speak, was using her movement to communicate. She—like anybody else in the world—wanted connection and this was her rather threatening way to get it.

I sympathized…and I didn't, too. The rooms she bounced around in were usually empty, and this was an eight-person group home! Before she had arrived, a group of residents usually gathered around, wanting attention from Ellen and me as soon as we walked into the house. One young man loved a tape of the old music TV show *Soul Train*. He would gesture in various ways to try to get us to watch it with him and notice what was going on. He was a fan and like any fan wanted to discuss it. Another resident knew us as friends of her parents and would come up to our faces, saying, "Mommy Daddy." She wanted to talk about them, about us, about our families, about whatever. Another resident would stand near us, smiling, saying a few things that we would try to stretch into a semblance of conversation, and we sometimes seemed to achieve this in a small way.

These were happy days when the group home felt like a small community and we felt part of it. But with Tracey's presence, those days were disappearing. It was easy to see why others didn't want to lounge on the couch and watch a show—Tracey would be in your face, with a stick, vaguely friendly and vaguely threatening at the same time. A couple of times I tried to sit with Walker and read something to him for a few moments, but Tracey would not let this happen. The moment we sat down she would be there, somehow between my eyes and the book I'd picked up. We'd ask the staff where everybody was and would get the answer that they were "upstairs in their rooms." The new implication was that the housemates liked to be alone. This was news to us.

Another good reason not to hang around the living/dining area was Brandon, the angry resident. Often we saw him sitting with a staff member, tearing paper into shreds. There used to be books and lamps and puzzle pieces lying on tables or chairs—signs of life and warmth and activities. Not anymore. It was clear that anything anybody was working on would fall victim to Brandon or Tracey. As time went by, no work-in-progress could ever be seen, along with table lamps or decoration for its own sake. The place became gradually less homey and more institutionally grim, more like a custodial care facility than a house where people grow, stretch, learn, and have fun.

The third new resident was Todd. In contrast to Tracey and Brandon, Todd was no danger to anyone. He was always to be seen at the front window of the house or at the window of the front door, sucking on a small towel, staring out and looking desperately sad. He had good reason to feel this way. Unable to move around without aid, and, of course, unable to communicate, he had no choice but to be stationary and alone. A staffer could stand by him and talk to him, and sometimes did, but no real exchange could take place.

Todd radiated sadness, something we knew could drive Walker nuts. Far from being the empathy-averse autistic of conventional psychological wisdom, it seemed to all of us that Walker was the emotion barometer of the house: he could tell if anyone was upset and quickly became upset himself. If I or Dave or Ellen was visibly unhappy, Walker would start laughing nervously and lightly push us. If, in a room full of laughing people, just one person was clearly miserable, this fact would be enough to upset him. Todd, just on the face of it, clearly needed something closer to a nursing facility—he couldn't participate in any active way in household activities: cleaning, doing laundry, cooking, making his bed, or being active in the vocational training program.

And, in turn, Walker must have driven the three new residents nuts. Tall, healthy, good-looking, and physically agile, with two smiling parents whisking him away every Saturday morning and breezing back Sunday afternoon, he must have represented everything that was out of reach for them. In taking him home, however, we weren't simply doing all we could for his welfare; we were also doing what was expected of us. In the original conception of the CILA, the idea was that families would stay together as much as possible and that weekends were a good time for the clients to be with their families. But not all clients, of course, were lucky enough to have this tidy nuclear family set-up. Some had only one active parent, and a few, such as Tracey, had no parent at all.

Indeed, none of the three new residents could participate in the vocational training program. Todd and Brandon would go to the center and merely sit. They couldn't begin to make an effort to have a stab at doing anything. They had to watch as others, like Walker, went out to jobs in a van while they themselves "failed" at doing this every day. And Tracey was too disruptive for the center. She was sent separately to another setting run by another organization, a special program where the emphasis was on sheer containment.

→ ←

And then, one by one, Walker's great friends began to leave.

The first was Nic. We always knew Nic was too good to last. His true friendship with Walker, his talent for understanding Walker as a real young man who wanted what other young men wanted, was a very rare thing. He seemed to have a secret line of communication with the normal guy behind autism's screen. But Nic was clearly a star in the making, a performer with a career ahead of him. Perhaps some of his talent for creating characters on stage was based on an innate ability to read people, an empathy for other people's point of view. *Something* powered his knack for truly *getting* our guy. After a farewell dinner with him at his choice of restaurant—the kind of out-of-the-way, cutting-edge cool place patronized by Nic's fellow tribespeople, all of whom looked as if they'd just stepped out of the artist's loft for a quick bite—Ellen and I tried to reassure ourselves that Walker still had friends at voc and at his house who knew him well.

But the key friend we focused on was also soon to be gone. Caroline, the supervisor of the house and Walker's special pal, was a short-timer too. And it was from Caroline that we received our first inklings of a connection between Walker's CILA life and his sleeping problem at home.

She told Ellen a story that was heartwarming and not so heartwarming at the same time. Early one morning Walker got up before everyone else and went down to the kitchen. Caroline was there getting the remote beginnings of breakfast ready. "Coffee?" Walker said.

Somewhat shocked for three reasons—(1) she'd never heard him say the word before; (2) she'd never known him to like coffee; (3) she'd never heard him suggest such a *social* activity—she set to work helping him prepare it himself. She was surprised how little prompting was needed, not knowing that he'd seen his dad do it every morning of his pre-CILA life. She also didn't know that "coffee" was a key term in his dad's Advice About Life. I used to tell him that coffee was a time-honored way to a woman's heart, that "having coffee" was what us guys did to get to know girls. He'd been to Starbucks a thousand times and normally had hot chocolate, but he knew this was not the real thing. "Coffee" was a word with some magic in it.

They then sat across the table from each other and sipped their cups in silence. (Or, rather, she probably sipped and Walker probably guzzled.) For a blissful moment they weren't caregiver and client, staffer and resident; they were two friends, Jennifer Lawrence and Bradley Cooper, sharing a moment. Suddenly, the spell was broken in a most un-Hollywood way. There was a commotion outside the kitchen. Caroline jumped up and dashed out: a resident had defecated on the dining-room floor.

Caroline related all this to Ellen and added a postscript: later that day, for no reason at all anybody could decipher, Walker pushed Caroline. Ellen said, "Well, he was mad at you for the incident in the morning, taking off in the middle of your coffee date."

"Yes!" Caroline said. "That's it. Yes, that's got to be it."

Caroline was our friend, but she was also an employee of the CILA. She had a certain loyalty to us, her friends, but she also had to watch her professional side. She couldn't tell us who slammed the door on Walker's little moment, but we knew because we'd seen her in action: Tracey. We knew too that cleanliness, order, and safety were the *sine qua non* of life at a group home. If three residents made these three issues the only things that could matter, well, then, those are the main issues

of the place. Everything else—growth, fun, even good cheer—
came second if these three criteria weren't met.

And the story itself had a backdrop: Walker had shoved
Caroline "for no reason." This was to become a refrain as time
went by and new staff came to the home. Walker did aggressive
things that seemed to come from, well, his own aggressive
nature. There was never a *cause* or *context*. There were never
any circumstances, any situations, that led to him shoving a
staffer. His actions sprang mysteriously from his own hostile
heart. Life in the CILA was perfect, according to the newer
staff. Any trouble came from uncaused misbehavior. In the case
of this story, it truly hadn't occurred to Caroline what Walker's
motives were. When Ellen pointed out her little deduction,
Caroline readily admitted the cause. Or maybe the story itself
was Caroline's cryptic way of letting us know: after all, she had
given us enough information for us to figure it out.

According to privacy laws, staffers were not supposed to tell
us which resident had done something dangerous or aggressive,
something that called for a staffer to write up an "incident
report." If one of Walker's housemates hit him and caused a
bruise—something that started to happen with increasing
frequency after the introduction of Brandon and Tracey—staff
were forbidden by law to tell us who had done it to him. These
strictures made sense. But they also fostered a defensive ethos
for the staff and the agency itself. The character—the purpose
even—of Walker's house was changing, but the reasons for
the change, even the fact that change was occurring, could be
hidden from parents or legal guardians. And hiding the name
of a client—a good and normal thing—came to slip over into
hiding circumstances. Because Walker could not speak—
indeed, no resident of the house could rebut anything said

about them—parents and guardians had to take the word of the staff. There was literally no one to contradict them.

→ ←

It became clear to us that Caroline was very unhappy with the way the group home was changing. She was the "boss," in a way, but she had no control over which clients were taken in or how the priorities of the place changed as a result. When Caroline announced that she was leaving to pursue graduate work in occupational therapy, we thought, *Well, of course. She's smart and ambitious and very talented at this work and feels despairing about creating a nurturing environment for her young clients.*

But, like a Hollywood movie cop with two weeks to go until retirement, she couldn't escape without big trouble.

We got a call one afternoon from the CILA. Could we take Caroline to the emergency room? She seemed to have suffered a concussion. So I raced to Walker's house and picked her up. On the way, I tried delicately to probe about how it had happened. Even in her rather dazed state, however, she could only tell me a client had hit her—had head-butted her, I assumed. It couldn't have been Walker, because the legal guardian was always notified in these cases. Caroline had suffered a concussion in a bike accident the year before, and she was very worried that this incident may have dangerously exacerbated the damage from that experience.

It did. Her recovery was difficult and she was concerned about her ability to handle class work. When she started graduate school the following fall, she was indeed like a "special" student who had to be allowed extra time to write exams. Her mental abilities were as strong as ever, and she passed all her classes, but there was a time lag in her thought processes. She knew that the brain damage might follow her all her life.

→ ←

Ellen and I were sitting in a North Side coffee house talking to our friend Pam, sipping lattes, eating pumpkin bread, and trying not to sound like monster fascist yuppie parents. Pam (again, not her actual name) was one of the main reasons we hadn't begun looking for a new residence for Walker as soon as the three new troublesome residents moved in. She was one of the directors of the agency, had known Walker for seven years, and had been there at the creation of the CILA and the voc program. Like Nic and Anastasia and Caroline, she had a gift for seeing more than "the autistic" in Walker. She knew, we believed, how important it was to continue the terrific vibe that the early CILA had, the feeling of a healthy, happy fraternity house that Doug had fostered.

We were going to ask her if maybe, perhaps, possibly, conceivably, Brandon, Todd, and Tracey could *move*—that is, *live in another group home created by the agency*—that is, *perchance*? We knew what this request would sound like; we knew it better than most parents. We'd heard it said or implied all of Walker's life, beginning with a comment Ellen picked up at a preschool introductory open house. She was holding the hand, very tightly, of a starry-eyed, hopeful but ultra-hyperactive four-year-old Walker and trying to make chit-chat. Nearby, a teacher nodded in Walker's direction and said to a mother, quietly but audibly, "Don't worry. He wouldn't last a week here." It seemed to us that the CILA used to be a rare place where low-functioning housemates were thriving. Now, because it seemed to be not selective at all about admitting residents, something precious had been lost. And our boy Walker could become a casualty.

Somehow we pitched our meek suggestion to her, and to our relief Pam completely agreed. Yes, of course, she saw the problem and shared our utter dismay. She explained that because the agency was becoming financially strapped, they had to take any client who applied. But she, Pam, would make sure the situation changed. She was already seeking other, more appropriate places for what she would later, angrily, term "the three Bozos" to live. She shared our disappointment with Walker's group-home situation, and she was determined to change it.

Our friendship with Pam was one reason we did not separate Walker from his group home. But the most important reason was that there was nowhere else to go. We believed we had no other options. Facilities for adults with disabilities were shockingly limited in Illinois. In our own exploration of group-home options, Ellen and I were put off by what we saw and read about. Newspapers sounded a steady drumbeat of stories of abuse and neglect in small group homes. And the putatively "good" group homes and vocational programs had waiting lists that would take Walker into his thirties or forties before an opening would appear—if ever.

Our only real hope was that change could happen.

CHAPTER 8

A Very Un-Merry
Birthday

AS I SAT AT the meeting, I wondered about my blood
pressure. Maybe what I was hearing required heavier cardiac
medications than the ones I was taking. Maybe some strong
anti-anxiety med should be added to the growing battery of
youngish-senior-citizen pharmaceuticals that I ingested each
day. The people around me at the table were all smiling and
super-agreeable, I knew, and yet I was feeling defensive, even
attacked. Ellen, of course, was sailing along with them on gentle
waves of goodwill. *Maybe I'm just crazy*, I thought—not for the
first time.

What I later came to think of as the famous Ominous
Staffing had started quite well. This was an Individual Service
Plan (ISP) conference, a "staffing," the occasion for the agency
employees to report to the parent or legal guardian of a client
on how things were going. I was attending this meeting because
I had always had a good record of friendliness with the staff of
Walker's voc program and group home and thus Ellen could
trust me to, well, *behave* myself.

Not so with Dave's staffings. Dave had always had an IEP, an Individual Educational Program. He read, did math and science, accumulated facts about the world, came up with questions and observations that were way, way above his so-called "grade level." He wrote songs, poems, essays, stories, drew cartoons, made jokes, invented wild characters with story trajectories, and did all this almost compulsively. The trouble was, the creative juices poured out of him in a way teachers found disruptive to the peace and quiet of the classroom. He might literally stand up and walk around the room when an idea hit him. So a compromise was reached: he could leave any classroom whenever he wanted and sit in another room with a computer and do his work there.

This remarkable arrangement was reached with enormous difficulty over a period of several years and many meetings, none of which I, the father, ever actually attended. Ellen would come home from a confrontation and tell me what had transpired: what angry teacher A accused Dave of doing, how narrow-minded teacher B thought Dave should behave, why administrator C wanted Dave expelled. I would hit the roof and storm around and inform Ellen of "just what I'd tell that ignoramus." All of which disqualified me from attending any staffings. You don't bring a clown to the nuclear disarmament conference; there's just too much at stake. So, typically, Ellen—sometimes accompanied by Dave's therapist and father stand-in, Rich Arend—would face several people—administrators and teachers—across a table and negotiate. Ellen would employ her usual method of speaking softly and hinting at a big legal stick. Rich would back her up with the authority of psychological science. This strategy was a stupendous success.

→ ↞

But with Walker's people I was always Mr. Charm. I liked them and, I convinced myself, they liked me. I always felt waves of free-floating love at these meetings. What a marvelous world it is, I would muse, that all these good people are focused on one helpless person, my son, and are actively concerned about his well-being. I'd think of all the disabled children in the world—forgotten, ignored, or even despised—and how here, in this room, the opposite attitude was in play. One person who cannot speak up for himself has a small platoon of friends in addition to his careworn parents looking out for him and trying to improve his life.

When Ellen and I arrived, I took the Chair of Dominance at the narrow end of a long rectangular table. Though not in charge of the meeting by any means, I felt my position gave me a certain advantage, the way a talk-show host sits at a slightly higher elevation than the guests. Thus, I admit, I began the meeting feeling somewhat at odds with the group. After all, we were worried about the wild behavior of two of the new clients that we'd seen at Walker's group home and were concerned about the reasons for his sleeping problems.

Despite these misgivings, to me the staff sitting around the table were all friends with near-visible halos over their heads.

On the long side to my left sat Ellen and next to her, Tammy (I've changed the names of staff here), a teacher at the voc center. She was a large young woman with a bright, pretty face who always saw improvement in Walker's efforts at the voc center. She helped him with Facebook and computer games and devised exercises to encourage speech. On her left was Daryl, Walker's oldest friend and teacher, a fine role model.

Handsome and kindly, he was in his thirties and had kids of his own. He was a reassuring figure to Ellen and me: he knew Walker well and could interpret intelligently his sometimes difficult-to-interpret behavior. Although Walker was now out of our sight most of the time, we felt good that he spent time with Daryl, his old friend.

Across the table from Daryl was Debra, the new head of the CILA. We liked her on sight when she was a staff member before her promotion. She had a look that was the careful antithesis of what we had come to think of as the Education Type. She was a TV character actor from central casting, the one who Thinks Outside the Box: twenty-something with many tattoos, turquoise neon spiky hair, casual men's clothes. In the world of special ed, her look seemed to mark her as independent and down-to-earth. This was not what one wore to a school teacher's job interview. She had a relaxed, matter-of-fact way of talking and seemed supportive of Walker. But she was as yet an unknown: she hadn't been on the job long enough for us to get a true impression.

Finally, sitting at my right hand, both literally and metaphorically, was Pam. She was our rock, our anchor in the storm, our confidante, our friend. No matter what changes happened in Walker's situation, as long as Pam was there, we knew he had a friend, someone who knew exactly who he was, someone with his best interests at heart. Soft-spoken and kind-hearted, Pam was a warm person who was trying to maintain that dream of a grade A+ CILA we once had but which seemed to be slipping away from us.

Notably missing from this meeting was marvelous Doug, who had been "let go" for financial reasons when a new executive director was hired. People—friends—seemed to come and go at a dizzying rate.

Then, in short order, this collection of stained-glass figures started making me squirm in my chair. First up was Tammy. "Walker doesn't seem to be able to concentrate at all lately. He won't do Facebook with me and seems anxious all the time. He won't sit at the table with the others and doesn't seem to be able to focus."

"Yes, that's what I've noticed too," said Daryl. "And when we go out, he seems to want food all the time and won't stay on task. I had to stop taking him to his job at the restaurant because he kept stealing food out of the refrigerator. It's strange behavior for Walker. What have you noticed at home, Bob?"

"Well," I said, "he's pretty happy at home. We haven't seen the sort of trouble you describe at voc. He smiles and has a good time. But he has a lot of trouble sleeping on Saturday night. We write schedules for him and set a timer and try to steer him away from his food obsession. But the food demands are a problem, sure."

"What about when you go on walks? Does he go where you want to? Does he demand food?"

Here he hit me in a vulnerable spot. We had fallen into an unfortunate rigid trajectory on our walks, Walker and I. He resisted trying out new destinations on the L and walks through unfamiliar neighborhoods. There had developed an undeviating lurch from Dunkin' Donuts to Starbucks to Walgreens, and I knew we could do better—fewer treats, more flexibility—and I said so.

"Well, I could go on a walk with you and show you how to deal with him. We'd like the way you deal with him at home to match how we deal with him at the center."

Sub-surface alarms and flashing lights started to go off in my head. *He* wants to show *me* how to walk with my son? I, who have walked with him for 26 years and know him better than anyone else could?! Instantly, as could happen in situations like this, I thought of my father and his brothers, all of whom died of heart attacks in their forties. I was outdistancing them in the actuarial-table category—thanks to better cardiac care than they ever had—yet, who knows? I say these thoughts bounced invisibly beneath my facial map, but I can't be sure.

Of course, Ellen managed to keep on sailing pleasantly through this.

"Oh, thanks, Daryl. That's a really nice offer," she said.

"And I could come over to your house and observe how you interact on the weekends," he continued.

"Oh, Daryl, how nice. I don't think that will be necessary, but thanks!" Ellen said, serenely.

My mind raced: *Never mind, Daryl old buddy, how Walker would take the spectacle of you in our house, second-guessing and micro-managing his dad from moment to moment.* These or some such words throbbed in my frontal lobe as I strained to follow Ellen's lead and look grateful.

Then he said the would-be soothing sentence that reverberated in my memory every time I saw him after this day: "Don't worry, Bob and Ellen. We still like Walker. I'm sure this is just a temporary stage he's going through."

At this point in our son's life, after befriending him and us for years, he thinks we should worry about them "liking" Walker? "Liking" him was just an option? *And Daryl, if you decide you "don't like" him, what then?* The remark was like a hairline fracture in our relationship with the staff that only got wider and more displaced as the weeks and months wore on.

Then it was Debra's turn.

She spoke in flat tones without looking at us and began by praising Walker and saying what a charming and intelligent young man he was. I smiled and imagined my systolic blood pressure number dipping a bit. But then she developed the retro theme begun by Daryl.

"Walker does seem to need too many notes and schedules written down for him. We find that timers and lists don't work. We've dropped all that. And he's been stealing food from the refrigerator. His behavior at the CILA has not been good. Sometimes he pulls on staff and pushes them. Maybe if you brought him back here to sleep every Saturday night and then picked him up on Sunday, that would make him more acclimated to our routine here?" she offered. "And I'd be happy to come over to your house and help you deal with him."

Now I was of two minds about this. Yes, I very much did want to have him sleep in his own bed at the CILA on Saturday night. This new "enemy insomniac" Walker was wearing us down—we had basically to give up the habit of sleeping on Saturday night. But this new note about "behavior" was puzzling. It was a note we'd hear often from Debra as the months wore on. It would become clear that she regarded her role as mainly disciplinary and interpreted any challenging actions on Walker's part as "misbehavior," the way an elementary school teacher might. Her tattoos and her neon hair somehow started to look less, well, *winning*.

Clearly there was a new idea afoot: that Ellen and I were responsible for this new uncooperative, unteachable Walker, that his one and a half days home on the weekend were ruining him and disrupting life at the CILA. They wouldn't say it, but the clear implication was that his parents were, to use a retro word, "spoiling" him. A warning shot was being fired by our smiling friends around the table: Any troublesome behavior Walker exhibited at voc or at his home would be blamed on Ellen and me and our bad parenting.

Finally, Pam smiled and cheerfully summed up: Walker was becoming a problem at voc and his house, and staff members would come over to our house to teach us how to deal with him. She beamed at us her warmest smile and hugged Ellen. Ellen smiled too and hugged them all and thanked them for their wonderful help and advice, and I tried to shadow her gestures a bit and robotically say thank you. My good behavior was technically maintained.

But the red mist was descending. For the first time, we left an ISP meeting feeling *handled*, not lifted reassuringly by a gathering of saints.

In our post-mortem in the car, Ellen thanked me for my polite performance and reassured me that she was angry too. She stared ahead and said, "Something is very wrong here. Something has changed in a big way. Nobody's ever accused us of turning Walker into an unmanageable person before. We thought they were on the same page as us."

"Do you think they might be sort of getting back at us for saying that the three new residents in Walker's house don't belong there? We've never questioned anything the agency did before. Maybe they feel that we're criticizing them," I said. "Or am I being paranoid?"

I was steering the car through the narrow streets and hit a speed bump a little too fast. The resulting jolt seemed to call to mind a vivid memory, one I'd tried to suppress with every bit of talent for avoiding the truth I could muster. It was though I had a denial app on my forehead that I tapped every morning as a defensive gesture to get through the day. This day I must have forgotten.

"Remember the birthday party?" I said.

Ellen looked at me. "Yes, I know," she said with a slight move of her head that said, *Let's not talk about that right now.* Ellen too was in denial about the quite un-merry birthday party of the previous December and all it suggested about what Walker was living through right now. But we both knew it was, in a way, the most critically important thing for us to keep in mind.

"But Pam already told me that she's working on moving the three of them. She said that they would live in another house the agency owned. Something must be holding up the process."

→ ←

Walker's 26th birthday had been different from all his others.

There had been lovely birthdays when Walker was very young: just the four of us family members around the dining-room table, streamers and balloons overhead, Walker blowing out his candles and all singing "Happy Birthday."

There had been troubled birthdays, too: two or three friends invited over for a celebration, but Walker so agitated or upset or frustrated that the guests had to leave early with hasty apologies from us about the unpredictable circumstances. "Sorry, guys. Sometimes it's just all too much for Walker," we'd say, grinning, as we hurried them out the door.

But there was never a birthday without a distinct undertone of alarm for Ellen and me. (And for Dave, too: after about Walker Birthday #4, he couldn't handle his emotions during "Happy Birthday" and he opted to stay in his room for the group sing.) Each passing year became a marker of how far

Walker was veering from the Normal Path. At ages three, four, and five he presented enough intelligence and competence to let us attribute much of his behavior to eccentricity. Every bell curve has to have its outliers, right? At ages six, seven, and eight, however, he was far, far off the Path. We were possessed of fierce hope about his future and bright determination to live in the moment—what a tragedy it would be, we'd tell ourselves, to let anxiety overwhelm the here and now—but the still, small note of terror had a way of breaking through. Something about the number of candles on the cake called up memories of ourselves at those ages, of the friendships and dreams and fun we'd had, that made our hearts ache about how much Walker was missing. Then, too, there were the unavoidable comparisons: Friend X's kid at this age was writing essays. Friend Y's little girl was nailing piano recitals. And what did Walker himself know about where he was on the great developmental curve of life?

I don't know much about the developmental curve, Dad, but I know how I felt on my birthdays and I was sometimes very happy and sometimes pretty disappointed. I love birthdays and birthday parties. I have a good memory and always remember special days and holidays. My birthday is always right after Thanksgiving and right before the Christmas season. It's the best time of year. Sometimes you and Mom made a big deal out of a birthday party, but sometimes you just kind of let it slide by. I loved it when you invited people over to the house and I know I sometimes couldn't handle that. Just like Dave, I get too excited. I go up and over when people get real emotional. Once Dave got under the table when we were singing and I kind of wanted to do that too. I don't think I worry about my future in any special way on the day of my birthday, though, because I always worry about it. I know I've got autism and am very different from others my age. I know because you've talked to me about it, but not very much really. Mainly—for just about my whole life—you've talked about it in front of me just as if I wasn't even there. I feel like an expert!

But the alarm of his 26th birthday was no undertone. It was more like an air-raid siren.

The event started out promisingly. Debra, then a new staff member, phoned us with a proposal. Maybe Ellen and I could bring a special birthday dinner over to the CILA for Walker and we could all celebrate there. Although the staff had often invited us over to have dinner with the residents, we'd never actually done it because we knew what would happen: the very sight of us at the house would make Walker itch to get out and into the car with us and go on the lam to have fun. It had happened at all events—picnics, parent conferences, parties; he'd immediately lobby strenuously to get going. But Debra was insistent that we should have a little dinner with all of Walker's housemates on his birthday, so we set the date.

On the day we drove to the voc center and picked him up after his work ended. We thought we'd run some errands (always a popular thing to do) and the last stop would be that finest of all fine dining experiences, the crème de la crème of magical moments in life: Kentucky Fried Chicken. First we went to what we'd come to call "the Happiest Place on Earth," the Lincolnwood Town Center Mall. We knew that the Disney company had claimed that title for Disney World and knew this claim to be, arguably, justified. Even though every single Disney animated film had a special place in Walker's heart due to repeated viewings of videotapes—"repeated" like a pneumatic hammer into his father's brain—both Walker and Dave had no interest in going to the place. Dave announced to us early on that he was afraid of the humans-dressed-up-as-cartoon-characters that roamed the park. He'd seen one such actor at the zoo and that was enough for him. Walker, who clearly could have let us know one way or another if a trip to Florida would be a treat, never so much as smiled when the prospect was laid before him.

But Disney videos throbbed in his head, and one spot in one film—the Mad Hatter's "Unbirthday Song" in *Alice in Wonderland*—was special to him—special to the point of obsession. He would wait for the scene, watching the movie in his calm but kinetic way, smiling and walking toward the TV screen and then backing up, waving his arms. When the Mad Hatter introduces Alice to the party at the table, he'd become very still and put his fingers in his ears as though something grand was about to take place. Then, as the song ended, he'd lose it: shouting and crying and insisting on seeing it again. In a house where rerunning videos was a way of life, a complete ban on this one had to be enacted, if only for the sanity of the family.

Why was this scene unique? It seemed to us that the party itself was the main thing for him: all that fun, all that wacky singing. Birthday *presents*, the main focus of a birthday for so many children, never seemed to mean anything to Walker. Every year it was a struggle just to get him to open the wrappers, and he'd usually set the game or puzzle or book to the side right away. Rather, what he loved had to be the celebration, the humor, the friendship. The scene was a signal to his mother and father that—duh!—the boy might love his own birthday in a special way.

After the excursion to the mall, where he strutted with a huge smile as though he was owner of all he surveyed, we stopped at Jewel to pick up a birthday cake and finally at Kentucky Fried Chicken. This was a castle located on a mountain top surrounded by trumpeting angels—at least one would conclude as much from the jumping-out-of-his-socks grin that Walker sported all the way into the place and out of it back to the car.

We had cake, we had birthday boy, we had buckets of chicken. But we weren't actually *ready*.

It began peacefully but oddly. Walker set the table, putting out paper plates and forks and napkins and then sitting down at the head of the table, Mad Hatter-wise. On his immediate right sat furious Brandon with a staff member ominously standing behind him, guard-like, rather than sitting next to him. To Brandon's right was sad Todd, and next to him an aide to help him eat. Next to Todd was familiar Steve, the only friend of Walker from the early days of the CILA, a gentle and pleasant nonverbal young man about Walker's age. Next around the corner of the table was beringed Debra assisting unpredictable Tracey. Next to Tracey was hopeful Ellen and finally me, a big wild-card Bob.

Our first question: "Where are the others?" Here were the three newcomers plus Steve, but where were the three other familiar figures we knew? "Oh, one is with her parents tonight and the other two are upstairs in their rooms. They already ate," was Debra's answer.

Next question, but unasked: *Is this how you normally have a party? Or a dinner? With a staff member standing guard or assisting each resident around the table?* We knew they had recruited at least two people part-time for this event, for there was nothing like one-on-one staffing normally in the house. This was clearly a special event, a planned party, because outside eyes—parents—were present. It was a special treat, clearly, and the staff wanted it to go well.

But nothing went well, actually. Brandon glared, tensely and menacingly, at Walker. The guard made sure that his hand never left Brandon's shoulder, at the ready to block any rapid moves. Tracey had trouble sitting at all and walked back and forth, making shrieking sounds behind Ellen and me. When she did eventually sit, she put her face down into her plate. Walker, no smiles anymore and looking very nervous, took only a bite or two of his chicken and then wanted to go up to his bedroom.

So Ellen and I spent the minutes at the table trying to coax, beg, tease Walker into staying there—to eat his favorite treat! When that was a lost cause, we introduced the birthday cake and the song. Walker blew out the candles and then pushed to leave again, without eating a piece. This was my son, the great gourmand, the omnivore! All the while Tracey was doing everything she could—making noise, moving around, playing with food, putting her head, face down, into her plate—to get attention. Todd poked sadly at his food. Steve ate readily, on his own island of silence. Brandon looked angrily at Walker and Walker's food. No treat, no bribe in heaven or on earth would be enough to get the party host to stay in this room. I couldn't keep Walker here any longer. On about his fifth try to get up and leave, I just let him run upstairs to his room.

I knew, guiltily, deep in my bones, that I felt exactly as Walker did. *I* loved fried chicken. *I* loved chocolate cake. But *I* wanted to get out of that room as fast as I could. My only thought, about five minutes into this party, was *Aren't we about done now?* I rehearsed excuses frantically in my head: *Ha, ha, don't I have papers to grade at home...? I think I'm getting a migraine... I need to sort my socks.*

Ellen and I, back in the car, tried to breathe again but respiration was second to guilt: *This is how Walker lives? This is what dinner looks like in his house? This is how he relates to his housemates? This is the best we can do for him?* These topics swirled in the air between us for hours afterward. But we kept coming back to three facts: (1) Our good friend Pam promised to move the three new residents. (2) We were still active at the agency and we believed we were in a position to change things. (3) There was nowhere else, no plausible place in the state of Illinois for Walker.

But we knew this house was no longer in the A range. Even if we graded on a curve, we were looking at a D.

→ ←

The memory of this real-life Mad Hatter party scene faded somewhat in the next few months. Ellen exchanged frequent emails with Pam, urging her, begging her to change the situation in the group home. Pam always insisted that any day the situation would change. But our contact with the reality of Walker's life at the CILA narrowed again to what it usually had been: the anodyne glimpses we had of it when we picked him up and took him back on the weekends. These glimpses themselves were sometimes revealing, but they allowed that party scene to fade until the picture was revived by the Ominous Staffing meeting where Daryl, Debra *et al.* offered to teach us how to relate to our son properly.

From that meeting on, however, the alarm bells never stopped ringing in our ears.

CHAPTER 9

"People Change"

"LOOK AT HIM," ELLEN whispered to me. "It's like he's got a sure spot on a flight out of Saigon." This was absolutely true, I thought. We'd just seen a documentary on TV the night before about the end of the Vietnam War and fresh in our minds was the footage of people wildly trying to escape. Walker looked as if he had just gotten the final seat on the last helicopter.

It was a stupendously weird place for him to be so happy and relaxed. We were in the waiting room of the University of Illinois Hospital emergency room, and had been sitting on the plastic chairs and pacing the linoleum floor for the last ten hours. It was 9 p.m. Walker hadn't had any of his usual treats. The battery of his iPad, on which he'd been watching his favorite videos, had been dead since six o'clock. He held in his fist a pile of index cards, on both sides of which his parents, the filthy liars, had written a sequence: "First, wait a little while. Next, the doctor will see you. Next, you'll go to a hospital room. Next, you'll get some pills to help you feel better." It was a situation that should have elicited every fiber of frustration in his body, and yet here he was: peaceful, smiling, quiet, cheerfully expectant.

We were there because Debra, the head of the CILA, had called to say that they were going to take him to the psych ward. The nurse for the clients in the home (she had become Nurse Ratched in Hughes marital parlance) agreed with her: Walker was wild, unmanageable, a "danger to himself and others." He needed a thorough psychological exam and better controlling drugs.

We were skeptical. An escalating cold war had been taking place between us parents and the CILA about Walker's behavior. Much that we were hearing about him seemed exaggerated and improbable. Some phone calls from the staff described Walker as "choking" and "slapping" other residents, two things we knew he could never do. When Walker was extremely frustrated, he could pull hard on someone, he could even bite someone, he could shout very loudly and push pretty hard, but he was a lousy fighter. Punching and slapping and choking were aggressive, fight-precise moves for the neurotypical community, not him.

But we also knew that Debra might have a point. Ellen and I had seen Walker in the state Debra described. He had been hospitalized in psych units three times in his life for "psychotic episodes." Once he had to be dragged from the waiting room into the examining room by hospital security. Once, when he was a tall teenager, Ellen and I found ourselves literally sitting on him at three o'clock in the morning just to control him as we stared into each other's eyes, baffled and frantic about what to do next. We knew Walker when he became terrified, and we knew we should be the ones to take him to the hospital.

On getting to the ER desk, we tried to explain that Walker, like many others with autism, could not wait, that he was likely to be a big problem in the waiting room. As with many such trips to hospitals, the nurse said, "Sure. It won't be long." But of course it was long—interminable, endless, unremitting, perpetual. Eleven o'clock became twelve, one o'clock became two, etc., etc. A line from Raymond Chandler always occurred to me in waiting rooms: "Another army of sluggish minutes passed by." Sluggish but anxious too: no matter how self-possessed Walker seemed, at any minute he might panic and waiting could become a crazy wrestling match.

The puzzling thing was that no wrestling match erupted then or for the next ten days that he was in the hospital.

→ ←

Months before this trip to the ER, phone calls from the CILA about Walker's behavior became more and more frequent. A staff member, usually Debra, would tell us that he had to be "written up" in an "incident report." Always, *always*, his eruptions were reported as completely baseless. Things in the house were tranquil and happy and then Walker—for no reason at all!—would attack someone. These calls were normally to our landline, not our cell phones. Gradually I got into a habit of waiting for Ellen to answer the home phone since I knew who it probably was. Once or twice I made the mistake of listening to Debra's tale of Walker's crimes and found myself getting into explosion mode. I would then hand the phone to Ellen, my stoic charm ambassador to the outside world.

Ellen's ability to listen to provoking, even hostile talk about Walker and not respond like her husband was limitless. I would sit, astonished, in our living room and stare at her while she spoke calmly, cheerfully, in an aren't-we-just-the-greatest-of-friends voice, while I boiled with rage. I was no more capable of responding that way to Debra's accusations than I was capable of tying my rigid baby-boomer frame into a pretzel like one of those Cirque de Soleil contortionists. At those moments Ellen seemed like a visitor from a better planet, one I was totally unfamiliar with. She knew, with the savvy of an experienced ambassador, that anger was weakness and more than weakness: it could cause the staff to ratchet up their dislike of Walker by proxy. He could become the one with the obnoxious parents, the one whose parents were the enemy, the one whose every misstep had to be amplified to prove a point. Ellen would probe, brightly, into the circumstances and always get the same response: Walker's behavior was "out of the blue" and had no context. And she would always apologize for him in a cool, measured way, then hang up in the same state of rage I was in.

Our good friend Pam had been behaving less and less like our good friend. Ellen was trying mightily to keep up the connection, to hang on to some sense of trust, but her efforts were proving fruitless. Pam continued to talk as though some other arrangement could be made for separating the three new residents—she still held out hope that Tracey, Todd, and Brandon could be moved to another house that the agency owned nearby. But she also started to tack off in Debra's direction about Walker, picking up the theme that he was "changing," becoming a "behavior problem." In one meeting over coffee, Ellen asked Pam why she thought these aggressive incidents were increasing in frequency. Then Ellen, the self-possessed charm ambassador, did *not* pick up her plastic tray and hit Pam over the head when she responded with these words and with a lightly dismissive gesture of the hand:

"Ellen, who knows? People change."

This remark burned in our brains intermittently in the months ahead. Whenever Pam expressed some retro idea about "them," how "they" do crazy and inexplicable things, this line—"People change"—flared up again.

We weren't used to this way of talking about our son. Previously, therapists and teachers—in fact, most staff at the agency—tried to scope out reasons why Walker or his classmates were doing apparently aggressive things. They would ask: What is the context of the behavior? What is the student trying to communicate? What have I been doing that might trigger this kind of response in the student? What signs have I missed that such a reaction was building? And the best question of all: What would I be feeling if I were *this* student in *this* situation right now? The best teachers and caregivers and friends of people with autism know a deep truth, one that flashes like a neon sign especially when things get rough: *Everything is communication.*

This truth puts a heavy—but also a highly interesting and challenging—burden on the teacher to *think.* Each autistic person has a special way of signaling his meaning, one that can differ wildly from one person to another. The teacher, like a World War II Bletchley Park codebreaker, has the job of deciphering what this word, that gesture, this look, and that repeated movement mean in such-and-such situation. It's a terribly demanding job, of course. It's one thing to calmly deduce that when Walker says "Shoes and socks," he means "I'd like to get out of here and take a walk." It's quite another to keep your composure when he does something world-shattering like shouting "Parmesan shining!" and tries to jump out of a moving car.

In Walker's case, "aggressive" behavior was sharply uncharacteristic. One incident stands out, one that was suggestive of his entire way of dealing with others. When he was about four, he was at a friend's house playing with her son, who was about three. Walker, always tall and strong for his age (his strength was a consequence of his constant movement), started shouting "Trouble! Trouble!" from another room. Whatever the problem was, Ellen's first elated thought was "My God! He's speaking!" Yelling for help using the correct word was something that, at that time and ever since, was a great rarity with him. When she rushed into the room, he was standing in the corner and the smaller, younger boy was hitting him as Walker stood there just crying and taking it.

Any aggressiveness on his part was always caused by fears bigger and odder than merely another kid attacking him. For example, the fatal getting up on a doctor's examining table. He had learned to like doctors and nurses very much over the years. By and large, they were kind and sweet with him, and he knew that they brought help for him to feel better. Our family doctor, Frank Weschler, was in fact a hero to him. But Walker couldn't bear the idea of lying supine on a table. It seemed to us that it seemed to him an insane abandonment of self-protection. So if anyone insisted that he even sit on this horrible table of sadistic torture, as Ellen and I and a nurse occasionally, foolishly, did, all hell broke loose. If pushed too far, he could pull and push and bite his way to the door to escape. Sometimes the doorknob of the examining room door itself became the locus of a crazy battle with parents and office personnel. It was fight *and* flight all the way.

But his passivity about personal attack became a worry after Tracey and Brandon arrived in the CILA. Sometimes he came home on the weekend with bruises. A round, fist-size mark on his chest? "We don't know what happened. We didn't see anything," was the staff response. A huge black eye? "He must have fallen out of bed." But on to his bedroom's carpeted floor? "Nobody saw anything. He must have hurt himself somehow."

Bruises on his upper body became common: on his back, on his stomach, on his neck and *nobody ever saw anything.*

The worst was the hand injury. He came home from the CILA one day with small marks above his wrist and a swollen, red hand down to very white fingertips. The doctor said the marks looked like small fingernail indentations. No bones broken, but Walker had a MRSA infection. Ellen quizzed an uninterested Pam:

> E: How did this happen?
>
> P: Oh, these things happen sometimes. He must have hit his hand on something.
>
> E: You mean he slapped something with the back of his hand?
>
> P: Probably.
>
> E: Don't those look like fingernail marks, as if someone had dug their fingers into his arm?
>
> P: No, they don't look like fingernail marks to me.

These, of course, are the answers of an organization circling its wagons: *Nothing can be wrong with the way we do things. Any problem must be the client's fault.* But Pam and the staff had had such a fine history of caring for Walker, of being protective and even loving, that we were reluctant to press the issue. Also, at the back of our minds, and sometimes right out in front, was the horrible fact of Illinois life that there was probably nowhere else to go. Walker was lucky to have a CILA at all, even one with a grade of D. He was over 22 and had a placement, for God's sake. He even had a vocational program. He wasn't on a thousand-person waiting list for a prominent group home. Why, we had hit the jackpot!

→ ←

A couple of months before the visit to the psych ward, Walker had his criminal trial. Of course, it was not meant as a "trial" at all. It was a conference of helpful professionals who had observed Walker carefully and had suggestions about how he might better be helped. But Ellen and I were wary and nervous about it. We had received so many calls about his "behavior" and the "write-ups" of his "incident reports" that we felt on notice and on our guard. With each call from Debra, who increasingly seemed to me more like a parole officer ticking off violations than a caring professional, we felt as of they were building a case against him. In fact, this phrase, "building a case," popped up with great frequency after every call from her, as in this slice of dialogue:

"What do you think's going on?" Ellen or I would ask.

"Well, obviously they're building a case," I or Ellen would answer.

"But why? To what end?"

"They want to kick him out of there. Or give him more drugs."

"But he's such a sweet guy. Why would they want to do that?"

"Because they're clueless and dumb. They don't know what they're doing," Ellen might answer.

"Because they're fucking assholes!" I might offer, helpfully.

The critical difference of this meeting was that the agency had called in two social workers from a group called the Hope Institute to observe Walker, both at the group home and at the vocational center. These two would write a report with analysis of Walker's situation and make suggestions about how it could improve. *Oh, sure,* we thought. *They've brought in people they could steer to their foregone conclusion that Walker needs more controlling medications or a more restrictive environment in some other—any other—place.* These were the two solutions we most feared.

We sat at the dining-room table of the CILA with the two social workers, April and Mary, and the usual suspects—Pam, Daryl, and Debra, this time sporting a new tattoo on her neck and neon green hair. I was preparing myself for the worst: (1) the representatives from Hope had drunk the agency Kool Aid, and so would take the agency line about how Walker was mysteriously turning into a dangerous character; and (2) I must *not* make a fool of myself. Ellen's voice had become higher, her reaction when she was very tired or very nervous.

After the introductions, Mary, the main social worker, spoke: "Well, we've looked at Walker a long time and what he basically needs, the underlying thing here, is that he needs to have more fun." Ellen and I nearly fell backward in our chairs. It was as if, instead of a sentence of hard labor, Walker was going to get a medal. The Women from Hope had put the blame, essentially, on the agency: Walker's needs were not being met. When we recovered, however, they did present a sad picture of a sad guy: uncooperative at voc and in the house, easily distracted from tasks, preferring to be alone in his room, prone to outbursts. It was not the Walker we knew at home; it was his CILA self—an obviously unhappy young man.

Their main recommendation was that Walker should have a one-on-one aide, somebody to go out with him on long walks, somebody who could take him to interesting spots in the city. Mary and April had observed the obvious: Walker was different from the three new residents, around whom the life of the CILA now revolved. He *expected* something out of life. He *expected things to happen.* He wasn't content with custodial care. Tracey, Todd, and Brandon never showed any desire to go anywhere or do anything. They had no interests, per se. And the other residents of the house were generally not visible, for they were upstairs in their rooms. We knew that it wasn't April and Mary's job to critique the group home or the voc center; their job was to intervene in the case of an individual—what they called "crisis intervention."

We thought maybe this would help. Maybe an aide— especially a smart, interested aide—would be the answer, we thought, and we went away from the meeting encouraged. But the wariness never let up; it was a new way of life.

→ ←

That summer Ellen and I devised a daring plan for an actual, but very small, vacation with Dave. We had never done this before. With just one exception, every family trip meant every member of the family piled into the car. That one exception had been the summer before when we took Walker alone on a trip to see relatives in southern Ohio. Dave had made it clear that he didn't want to spend that much time driving with his brother, and we sympathized entirely. At some point, Dave deserved to not have the stress of being with Walker.

Normally, the full-family road trip went like this: Walker demands to stop at every interstate rest area, whether a bathroom break is needed or not. Walker has trouble sleeping in the motel, sometimes staying awake all through the night, keeping the rest of us awake. When we visited the homes of friends and relatives, Walker's internal timer of tolerance generally rang after a half hour's visit. Then I would take him for a ride in the car while Ellen and Dave stayed behind for a predetermined length of time, say an hour. No matter what Dave did or where Dave went on this "vacation," Walker's timer of tolerance ticked away, limiting the minutes spent doing anything at all. Fishing, boating, swimming, hanging out with good friends—any activity—was limited by how long Dave's brother could stand to do it. When they were both younger, it hadn't been this way. Walker could exist happily in almost any place indefinitely. But as time went by, his ability comfortably *to be*, *to exist* in the house almost completely vanished. Why? Why did so many things he once did, and did enthusiastically—ice skating, ball playing, swimming—fall by the wayside as he got older? There were a thousand questions that banged frustratingly around in my mind about autism. The great god Medical Science had nothing to say about these or any of my other questions.

The previous summer we let Dave stay home while we took Walker to Ohio to visit our friends. It was a Well-Meaning Experiment. Maybe Walker would like to have us all to himself. Maybe he'd enjoy getting out of town. He had been suggesting "Ohio! Ohio!" recently and we thought it would be a treat. After nine hours of driving, we checked into a motel in Ellen's home town in southern Ohio, had an enormous pizza, and turned off the lights. But he stayed awake, on high alert, all night, looking through the curtains of the Holiday Inn at the parking lot, pressing us periodically to get back in the car. The next morning we stopped by our friends' house—a lovely house in the woods, as refreshingly different from our Chicago neighborhood as a place can be. But our nerves were shattered, our eyes bloodshot, and so we said hello/goodbye before driving back to Chicago. All the way, he shouted constantly to stop at rest areas and gas stations for Pepsis as we strained mightily, and sometimes failed spectacularly, to keep our tempers.

Ah! The good old Well-Meaning Experiment! Our philosophy was that one should try and *keep trying*, again and again, because one never knew when something might click with him. One should never, say, take Walker bowling and if he shows no interest, decide "Well, he doesn't like to bowl" and never go again. If that were the rule, life would systematically shut down for him. The growing list of nevers might crush life's possibilities. So the rule became "You never know!" This put the ball back in our court for us to keep in play. That's why we tried to take him to Ohio to repeat some good childhood memories. But sometimes this rule—how shall I put it?—just sucked.

But Dave, we decided, deserved a little trip without his brother. He, like Walker, loved long drives and seeing relatives in Ohio. His memories of the place were precious to him and this time he got to experience it all without counting the minutes until his brother couldn't stand it anymore. This time we rented a nice cabin on a secluded lake. We went fishing. We ate meals on a porch overlooking a lake. We had fun with our friends, Christy and John, who drove us through their woods on a hilltop in their little Jeep.

The trip was a miniature vision of what the normal families do. We learned again the meaning of "hanging out." We hung out with our friends, as in going to the county fair and taking in the cattle exhibits without nervously gauging how far the barn was from the parking lot in case Walker needed to make a quick exit. We said, "Hey, guys, want to go to a coffee shop or take a walk or just stay here and talk?"—and did this without looking over our shoulders. We listened to a gospel bluegrass group and ate hot dogs and talked about our families. We had three days of strolling, gazing, meandering, chatting, laughing: unhurried, untimed fun.

My habitual fatherly way of "being with" the family was pretty much to have an invisible blinking Walker monitor in my brain that perpetually told me where he was, what he was doing, how he was feeling. Ellen handled about 80 percent of the parenting work. My main job was physical Walker-wrangling. This meant that in social situations I was the designated parent, pal, therapist, gym coach, teacher, and safety officer for him.

This also meant that when Walker was present (most of the time for the first 21 years of his life), I was not fully "there for" Dave, as in "My dad was always there for me when I was growing up." This maddening sentence appeared often in my students' essays in Freshman Composition classes. I always winced when I read it, not just because the phrase was a cliché, but because I imagined Dave writing, "My Dad always imagined that he was there for me, but he wasn't, really." Oh, I was "there" all right; I was stapled to the living room most of the time. It was the "for" part that lacked reality. The awful truth was that early on in their lives I became, sort of, Walker's parent and Ellen became, sort of, Dave's. Times when Ellen connected well with Walker and I connected well with Dave were special to us, talked about, celebrated.

So this trip was one of those moments when the parenting equilibrium righted itself a bit, at least for me. But returning home would smash this illusion fast.

→ ←

The smash-up happened right away. We came back on a Thursday. On Friday morning we got the call from Debra: "Walker is unmanageable. We want to take him to the hospital and have him examined in the psych ward. The nurse says he needs more meds and we wonder if he's having seizures. She thinks he needs an EEG." Nurse Ratched was becoming very big on neurological diagnosis, a habit she would step up as time went by. We said that we'd be happy to do it, especially since the CILA was chronically understaffed. We even wondered—but quickly put the suspicion out of our heads—if they wanted him out *because* they were understaffed. So we took him to the UIC Hospital despite our misgivings about the idea. In his three previous stretches in psych wards, no new medical information was discovered, no solution to the mystery of our son was ever forthcoming.

It seemed that the tacit purpose of a psych ward was to give everybody a sort of enforced rest. The family had a break from the turmoil; the child had a—perhaps welcome?—break from the family. In the case of a group home and a resident, maybe the same brief sabbatical idea was the goal? But there was no grumpy Dr. House from television land at the hospital to zero in on the permanent puzzle Walker presented. On one notable occasion Walker was a difficult child going in and was exactly the same difficult child with the same very specific difficulties going out. Faced with a psychotic episode, however, Ellen and I ignored our principle that "nothing is accomplished in a psych ward" because, hey, there was nothing else we could do.

This case was different, of course. We had to take someone else's word for Walker's unmanageability and there was no claim that an actual psychotic episode was in progress. All we could do was report what Debra told us. And even in the waiting room, the sticking point was becoming evident: Walker, calm, smiling, cooperative, was showing no signs of the wild person we were there to describe.

→ ←

Who knew a psychiatric ward could be paradise? Certainly not Ellen and me. We'd been to them several times before and this floor was a seven on the depressing scale. But Walker took to the place like it was Club Med.

The décor was movie mental-patient grim. Linoleum floors, wide halls, a room with a closed blind that would not open, a table and one chair and a TV with a DVD player, and unhappy adult patients all around. There was also an aide stationed right in the room—a huge, strong African-American guy named Duane sitting near the door in front of a computer, there to quell the beast whose reputation had preceded him. But there was no beast, no trouble, no difficult young man yelling and pushing and trying to get out—just a cooperative, smiling young gentleman who couldn't tell anybody a thing about how he was feeling.

Later, we did understand, as clearly as if Walker could explain it to us.

How was I feeling? I could have sung the soundtrack of Mary Poppins, Dad. I was so happy to get away from voc and the CILA and be with you and Mom and the hospital staff. Duane was great. He talked to me like a real person. And you guys brought me my favorite McDonald's meals. It was fun to go to the lunch room and watch the big TV screen and eat with Duane and Charles and James—they were cool guys a little older than me and they liked movies too. It was fun to watch videos on the iPad. I was a big fan of Toby Keith back then and the song "Red Solo Cup" was always going in my head. I could breathe and relax and nobody was angry with me. And they gave me blood tests. I like those. I always feel like I'm getting better when I take those. I hated the EEG test, though. I can't stand those wires on my head.

→ ←

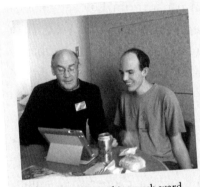

Walker and Dad in psych ward

Ellen and I were there for several hours each day of the ten-day stint. We spent a lot of time with the iPad, a lot of time writing things down on index cards, a lot of time talking to doctors and nurses and aides. Each day around 4 p.m. Walker would make it clear he wanted us to leave. He was enjoying his adult experience of being on his own with new friendly people around. One day he took my baseball cap off my head and put it on his own. Another day when we arrived, we walked in on a marvelous scene. There sat Walker in my baseball cap watching the film *Old School* with Duane.

Most films that Walker watched, even at age 27, were childish in one way or another. Disney cartoons and anything with the Muppets were his mainstays. We tried often to get him interested in live action, nearly adult fare—he learned to like the Indiana Jones movies, but never got into *Star Wars*—yet basically he shunned "adult" films or TV sitcoms or news or sports or talk shows. But Duane was *cool*. And Duane wanted to watch *Old School*, a very funny and profane movie featuring guys hanging out with other guys, having fun and being goofy—a feature film version, in a way, of Toby Keith's video "Red Solo Cup." Walker, we could see, was a guy hangin' with another guy, doing what guys might do in their man cave: watching Will Ferrell and Vince Vaughan and cracking up. *Could we adopt Duane?* I was thinking. *Would he want to live with us? What if we purchased the entire Will Ferrell DVD oeuvre?* We were clearly glimpsing a version of Walker we'd never seen before: a young man who wanted all the things a young man wants.

He was having fun, but he was also communicating: *This is what I want—a normal-ish world with friends*. Ellen and I were beginning to see Walker in a new way, but were even more despairing about how we could actually help him realize his wish.

The neurologist in charge knew Walker well. He had seen him in doctor visits numerous times. He could find nothing wrong with Walker—other than his autism, of course—and the EEG was normal. "He's the same charming guy I've always known," he said as Walker was leaving after the ten-day stay. "I don't really see the problem they see at his group home."

This was, of course, a very happy result, but somehow we knew it wasn't going to sit well with Debra and her medical backup, Nurse Ratched.

Chapter 10

Agitation: Father and Son

I WAS IN A hurry. It was a clear, sunny Saturday morning just after Walker's discharge from the hospital, and I needed to pick him up from the group home and get the car back to Ellen, who had an appointment in an hour. Kevin, a new staff member whom I'd never met, greeted me at the door. Ellen told me he was nice and attentive to Walker but warned me that he was on the fussy, supercilious end of the social spectrum. So I was in my most Friendly Dad mode. I greeted him with the best I could manage—my unimpressive version of a hearty handshake and smile—and told him I was sorry not to chat but had to move along. Walker, standing right next to him, was ready to go.

Then I remembered what I was supposed to check and, stooping to look at Walker's feet, said, "Uh-oh. He doesn't have on his special socks." These were expensive, difficult-to-don "therapy socks" his doctor had prescribed for his swollen ankles. Nurse Ratched insisted that the swelling was due to the lorazepam that the doctor had recently prescribed. It's a drug to quell anxiety. After doing extensive blood tests and eliminating other possibilities, our doctor suspected that Walker was malnourished. Like the unexplained bruises and swollen hand, this was yet another mysterious physical problem Walker was saddled with. Our doctor insisted that no, lorazepam couldn't possibly have that effect and prescribed therapeutically tight socks. (We later found that the nurse refused to give Walker the lorazepam, insisting on her diagnosis. Canceling the doctor's orders was to become a habit with her.) I asked Kevin for the socks and reassured him I'd put them on him when we got home because I knew that squeezing his big feet into the tight elastic was exhausting, irritating, and frustrating.

"It takes a village to get these socks on him and, of course, there's never a village around when you need one," I said, still smiling.

"What socks?" Kevin asked. A certain—I don't know—haughtiness was creeping into his tone. I explained: big, odd, tightly woven socks the doctor had prescribed for his ankles.

"Nobody told me about any socks," he said. Did he roll his eyes, or was I just slipping into Angry Dad mode? "Walker, why don't you go upstairs and look for your socks?"

"Oh, no, Kevin. That's not gonna work. He wouldn't be able to distinguish these new ones from his others."

"Walker needs to learn to follow directions, Mr. Hughes. We need to be patient and see what happens." From pretty extensive living with Walker, I could imagine what would ensue: Walker would go to his room and stay there. He'd need to be retrieved. Or he would go upstairs, then quickly come back empty-handed because he wanted to get going.

"This won't work," I said. "And I'm on a short leash from home right now, ha ha. I should go up to help him." I went upstairs and searched high and low for them. No socks. I came downstairs again with Walker.

Kevin said, "Why don't you go into the basement and see if they're in the laundry near the washer, Walker?"

"Oh, no. We won't have time to do that," I said.

Slowly and quietly, oozing condescension, Kevin pronounced, "Well, I can see where Walker gets his agitation."

→ ←

Angry Dad, of course, blossomed into being immediately, but he did manage to keep his mouth shut. Walker and I left, and I steamed in silence driving back home. *What's going on here?* I wondered. I'd never met Kevin before, and right away he's openly psychoanalyzing me. He seemed to be voicing an opinion he had picked up elsewhere. We knew that the CILA staff, via Nurse Ratched and Debra, did not like the "therapy socks" idea. They told Ellen that they thought the doctor had caused the swelling by prescribing lorazepam. They were bound to be very disappointed in the non-result of his stay in the hospital. In any case, malnourishment could point to something wrong with the group home, and that was not possible.

No one said it, but as the weeks went by it became clear that the nurse suspected that somehow, in some way, Ellen and I were manipulating Walker's doctor, even the staff at the hospital, into our pet Hughesian diagnoses. She began to insist that someone from the staff must be present at all of Walker's appointments.

Thus began what can only be described as a bizarre "cold shoulder" campaign instigated by the staff. Each employee of the group home, one by one, started to ignore us when we picked up Walker on Saturdays and dropped him off on Sundays. We would walk in, and where previously we'd exchange friendly greetings and jokes, we'd now be greeted by silence and averted eyes. On one occasion, Ellen rang the bell and could see Kevin through the window, staring at her, unmoving for a couple of minutes. She knocked on the door. He stared. This standoff went on for three minutes until another staff member opened the door. We would complain to Pam about the weird treatment we were getting, and she would either say we must be imagining it or that she'd talk to them about it.

Then, just three weeks after his stay in the psych ward, Nurse Ratched insisted that Walker go in again. His behavior now was extremely strange, she said. The staff reported that he would stay in the closet of his bedroom and refuse to leave all day (all day! And they hadn't called us?); that he would refuse to go to voc in the morning; that he'd refuse to eat; that he'd never talk, but merely grunt; that he would sit in the corner and cover his ears or stand and take his shoes off and put them back on again. Kevin sneeringly told me Walker had become "anti-social." (Spiky-haired Kevin, who had little experience and no education in special ed and yet who habitually spoke with the authoritative tone of the Surgeon General, seemed to actively dislike Walker.) The hitch was that they didn't want Ellen and me to "influence" the hospital staff. They insisted that our visits should be severely limited.

Nurse Ratched was the instigator behind this push to get Walker into the psych ward again. I, Bob, the short-fused avoider of confrontation, never actually spoke to the Ratch. Ellen described her as a gravelly-voiced, pugnacious bully on the telephone, an expert at putting people on the defensive. Neither of us had actually seen her. She was like a director invisibly barking instructions to the cast from somewhere off the stage. I knew that if I actually had to listen to her, I'd probably just start impotently shaking my fist at the phone, my lips moving but no actual sounds coming forth. This was the winning reaction I typically exhibited when discussing our credit card bills with bank personnel. Ellen knew this too and always answered the landline. She somehow managed to maintain the chipper tone, the cheerful attitude.

The nurse was convinced Walker had an underlying neurological problem that the Hugheses and their pet neurologist would not acknowledge. Walker, according to her, needed a CAT scan and an MRI. As Debra put it in a letter to the neurologist: "The staff and nurse are worried that there may be underlying neurological problems that we are unaware of." This message did not go down well with the doctor, the head of the neurological department of the hospital. He was basically being told that he had missed Walker's problem during the first hospital stay because he hadn't performed the necessary tests— that is, he hadn't done his job. After all, *the nurse and the staff agreed on this*!

→ ←

This would be a good point to explain something that I think might haunt some readers. The question is this: "Well, duh! How could Bob and Ellen keep their kid in such a deplorable place? He clearly is very, very unhappy. His health and safety are endangered. He's around people all day who either don't understand him or don't like him. The agency will not tell the truth about what goes on there. Why don't the parents pull him out of that place, for God's sake?"

This question was ours too, every day. And every day we came up with the same answer: *There's nowhere to go.*

At first we had hesitated because of our own emotional investment in the place. For one thing, we had friends there (though most had left or been let go). For another, we had been instrumental in establishing the home in the first place. And Ellen, in her work writing grants for the agency, had made a name for the program as a model for low-functioning autistic adults. Cutting and running was difficult; we kept hoping that we, powerful and active parents in our imaginations at least, could change things.

When this mirage evaporated, we were left with the fact of Illinois' miserable support for adults with disabilities. Politicians in the state who cut funding for health clinics and adult group homes are often lauded by newspapers for "having the courage to make the tough decisions." As I write, our current governor has targeted autism funding in particular for draconian cuts. Illinois isn't ancient Sparta, where disabled infants were left to die of exposure on hillsides, but some voters here seem to envy the practice.

But at this point, between psych ward stays, we realized Walker had to get out of there, one way or another.

Our good friend Pam, we had to admit to ourselves, was no longer a friend. She and others in charge had new agendas. For one thing, the funding for the agency was shaky and getting shakier. The state was very, very slow to pay its share of the expenses and the agency seemed incapable of or uninterested in approaching new funders for grants. And they were becoming short-staffed. Twice Ellen and I returned with Walker when there was no one in the house—no one at all: no resident, no staff member—but the door was open. We drove around with Walker and returned an hour later when a couple of staffers had finally arrived.

Under these conditions, a client like Walker—someone who expected to have fun and interesting jobs and novel experiences—was just trouble. Clients like the three newcomers, however, were comparatively easy. Custodial care always is. Tracey, for instance, could be left to freely run around the fenced-in yard or the living/dining area while the staff watched Netflix or sat on the porch busy with their smartphones. Walker and his parents, however, were in their faces, expecting something, anything, positive to happen. In Walker's first years there I always prefaced a proposal to take him home with "Of course, if there's anything planned here, I don't want to take him away from it." Often, there were outings and barbeques and games planned. In the last two years, however, I'd stopped asking. There were never any plans other than to hold the fort, sit still, and rely on the residents to stay quiet in their rooms.

Violent Brandon had lately become no problem. He was now, every time we entered the house, curled up in a fetal position, sucking his thumb and listlessly staring ahead. Rules forbade telling anyone about his condition, but clearly he was now heavily medicated, an easy solution for an understaffed group home. This seemed to be the plan the nurse had for Walker, too, but the parents and the neurologist were blocking the way.

The CILA's purpose was now mere custodial care because imaginative activity required money that the agency did not have. But instead of just leveling with us about the situation, Pam, the nurse, and the staff insisted on the Walker Has Mysteriously Changed narrative.

→ ←

So back into the hospital psych ward the eager Walker went. Now he was back with his friends; now he was in his element. You could see it in his face: this was *living*.

Ellen and I, now forbidden to hang out with him very long, would visit for just a couple of hours each day. There was no need to restrict us, however. This time Walker would take our hands and lead us to the door when he got tired of us. He was in his world now—it was none of our business. Who wants embarrassing parents to hang around the frat house?

His EEG turned out negative. The neurologist, now frustrated with the nurse's directions, refused to put Walker through the MRI gauntlet, certain nothing would turn up. Walker, as far as he was concerned, was a charming, cooperative, smiling young man with low-functioning autism. No show of wild aggression was forthcoming or even imaginable from this patient. Short of a Dr. Jekyll and Mr. Hyde potion, there was no medical explanation for the radical behavior shift. After another ten days in the hospital, Walker was released, again with a positive profile from the hospital.

The question, asked many different ways in conversations with many different people and in many different venues: "What's going on with him?"

> *Can I just put my two cents in here for a minute, Dad?*
>
> *All this talking! You and Mom and the doctors and the nurses and the group home staff and my teachers and plenty of other people talk and talk and talk—right in front of me like I'm not even there. It's very hard to take. I know you love me and all that, but it's really hard on me.*
>
> *Try to imagine that somebody stuffed a rag in your mouth and then started to ask you what was wrong. Or, still with*

the rag in your mouth, started to guess what your thoughts were in a group of people having a tense discussion about what you were thinking. Sometimes when you all are talking, I can't understand because I'm too upset and all the words are just a lot of noise. But usually I understand everything you're saying. One reason I didn't want Mom and you in the hospital was all this jabbering about me. You get between me and my friends. It's just not cool to be treated like a baby who can't talk.

Back at the group home and his voc program, the same story all over again. This time the staff at voc called us to say that Walker refused to participate at all in the activities. Instead, he started a new, almost Chaplin-esque routine. He would place a chair next to the door to the outside. He'd sit on the chair and take off his shoes and socks and put them on again, stand up and rattle the doorknob. Then he'd repeat this—*for hours.* Did we have any guesses about what the mime show meant? Ellen explained that—surprise, surprise—he probably wants to get out of the room.

"That can't be it," the staffer said. "Daryl took him for a walk around the block, but he's still doing it."

He doesn't want to take a walk. He wants out of the place, was what Ellen wanted to say but couldn't.

A week later, while I was teaching class, they called to report an emergency with him. He was violent, they said, he was hitting people, and we had to take him away. Ellen drove over and while she was trying to talk to Tammy, his teacher, Walker shouted and pulled away from everybody and ran into the street. Ellen and Tammy chased him but couldn't restrain him. "He's running away! See what we're talking about?" Tammy shouted as they struggled with him.

"He's not running away," Ellen shouted as drivers braked. "He saw our car parked across the street and wants to get in."

Ellen, gripping Walker as best she could, escorted him into our Honda. He slammed the door and locked it as he sat down, as if it were the world, not he, that was threateningly out of control.

"Do you need help in the car?" Tammy asked, the presumption being that he was now Mr. Hyde and Ellen would need SWAT team-level backup.

"No, he'll be fine with me. He's not going anywhere. The car is all he wants."

⇀ ⇌

This was the beginning of our new anxious and arduous lifestyle. Walker, they made it clear to us the next day, was out, permanently. We had to find a new place for him, preferably a group home or institution for violent individuals. The new arrangement was this: Walker could continue to sleep at the group home. This, as far as they were concerned, was a very generous concession. He had a good bedroom there to himself, more than he had in our house. But he would have to be picked up early in the morning and brought back by us around nine in the evening. It seemed quite necessary to me that he continue to sleep at the CILA. We needed to get sleep each night and couldn't get any with him so frequently awake. Besides, if he went too long without sleeping at the group home, the agency would lose funding for him.

Before this change, we would pick him up after the vocational program at three in the afternoon and bring him back to sleep in the CILA at nine. This permitted me to teach in the morning until 1:30 and be free to get out for our big walk in the afternoon. The one priority was to keep him away from the staff at the home as long as possible. But now that he was a public enemy at the voc program too, Ellen would have to pick him up each morning and occupy him until 1:30 when I could take over in the afternoon.

The two of us, both over 60, both with arthritic knees, now had custody of the violent criminal who could not be controlled by the young, healthy "experts" on the staff.

→ ←

On a brilliant mid-October afternoon, Walker and I turned on to Clark Street to go north for the last leg of our daily trek. This was the spot where each day, fittingly enough, I began to feel I was on my last legs too. My knee braces always started to fail me at this point, and my thoughts certainly did not match this stunner of a day. October is the best month to live in Chicago: the brisk air, the sky a deeper blue, the trees a Technicolor show, the street faces bright with energy.

But my mind was film noir all the way. Why was Walker so underweight? Lately, we had to devise strategies to get him to eat anything at all. In the span of a year, he had descended from a peak of 240 pounds, sped past his ideal weight of 195, and on to that day's worrisome 155 pounds. We compiled "food logs" and wrote down his meager intake for a day. Sample: "One hamburger, a can of V8, six French fries, half an ice-cream cone, most of a Coke." How could we get him to relax?

In the house, he was jittery all the time, asking us to "write stuff down" on index cards, his lists that reassured him that there really was a future, that the next three hours of living were real and wouldn't vanish as we all stepped forward into them. There was a good chance that he himself was worried too about his long-range future: What was going to happen to him? Where would he live? What would his days look like? His mom and dad had no idea and no ability to write these answers down on index cards.

This walk was the best moment of his day—pretty much the only good moment. Moving along in the city he loved was always a game changer for him. Somehow it cleared his head, set his mind at ease. So the two of us, hand in hand, walked quickly along, on his face a friendly smile, on mine, a what?—a "step-aside-stranger"-type glower?

I was self-absorbed and self-pitying, on the edge of snarling at innocent passersby. Then we halted at the "DON'T WALK" sign at Belden to witness a slice of traffic life that jolted me out of my mood. An attractive woman in her twenties, with long brown hair, red scarf, and fashionably torn jeans (an experienced observer of urban life, I can take in such details in a split second), was on a bike holding her hand out to turn left and waiting for the oncoming traffic to pass her by. A young man in a shiny new black Jeep behind her also wanted to turn left. I could discern this because he was blasting his horn over and over at her and inching his car toward her back tire. He was having none of this waiting-for-a-bicycle stuff! He was a guy! He had a Jeep!

But this is what really got me: the young woman had a *smile* on her face! It wasn't a passive-aggressive smirk; it was just an all-purpose smile at life. She was going to make a safe turn, and she was still enjoying the nice Chicago day.

The line of traffic kept coming and coming. The woman kept waiting and smiling. The driver of the Jeep would soon need defibrillation.

Suddenly, she turned around and, motioning with her hand, invited the driver to make his turn behind her. I could see right away that he liked this idea because he roared around her, nearly colliding with a car head-on. Then the young bicyclist, a philosopher-saint apparently, shook her head and smiled. It was a shake that said, "Oh, how silly people can be!" She then turned and went on her smiling way.

As the sign turned to "WALK" and Walker and I crossed the street hand in hand, I told myself, *Let this be a lesson to you, Bob. If you'd been on that bike, your head would have exploded with anger. Your blood would have boiled for a long time afterward. Your mind would have been a blur of goofy revenge fantasies. But here's this philosopher-saint sent to teach you something. Learn it!*

Braced by this new resolution, I let Walker lead me into Walgreens #2. The routine here was to let him go alone to the back of the store where the ice-cream cones were and get one for himself. It was a rare time when I stepped aside and let him just be a consumer on his own for a minute. Sometimes the routine had funny results. After a few minutes I'd see people emerge from the ice-cream aisle looking a little flustered or confused: this meant Walker must be having some trouble deciding what he wanted, opening and closing freezer doors and cheerfully getting into people's way. Then I'd have to retrieve him. But usually things went fine. We were known and liked by the clerks in the store. I always made a policy of chatting people up wherever we went and found that, by and large, clerks and salespeople were kind and understanding.

Today I wanted to buy more index cards. With Walker's new nervous state, we were burning through stacks of cards at a very rapid rate. The two of us walked over to another aisle and I spotted on a ragged tag underneath the display that the stacks of a hundred cards were two for one. Two for one! Oh happy day! In my tiny world, I had won the lottery.

We stood in a long line and Walker was pleasant and patient. The cashier, a new guy to me, rang up the cards but without the discount. I pointed out, in an offhand way as though it didn't really matter to me, that they were actually buy one, get one free. "No," he said. "There's no discount."

"Really, there is," I said, but knew I was stepping into dangerous emotional territory.

He looked at Walker and sized up the situation. "I'll go check." He was gone two minutes or so, and Walker's timer, I thought, might go off.

He returned and said, "Sorry. There's no discount."

Clearly, I was worried about the wrong timer here. I pulled poor Walker over to the stationery aisle, found the obscure sticker that announced my precious deal, could not get near the beleaguered cashier who was now overwhelmed with a staggering line of customers, and so found a manager who gave me my glorious, my stupendous, my precious steal of a deal.

This exhibition was not a good start for my new life as a philosopher-saint. But I decided: character, like Rome, wasn't built in a day. I tucked the girl-on-the-bike episode into my mental bank of Models for Living and hoped for the best.

I was going to need it.

CHAPTER 11

Psycho Dad Makes a Personal Appearance

ONE DAY IN THE winter of 1991 I decided I was having a heart attack. "Decided" is the key word here. Friends who have real heart attacks usually don't report that a decision was somehow arrived at regarding a cardiac catastrophe. Their stories employ terms like "shit!" and "my God!" and others indicating The End Seemed Near. So I went to the hospital for several days of tests only to discover that my heart was never in danger; after looking at my catheterization results, the doctor said, "There's not a person in this hospital who wouldn't be proud to have your arteries." *But maybe your brain, Mr. Hughes...* On being discharged, I left with a prescription for Xanax and a recommendation to try biofeedback techniques to relax.

What I had, in retrospect, was a predictable panic attack brought on by Walker's autism. And the four days in the hospital didn't help. Walker was a very difficult child to handle and an enforced four-day incarceration watching TV in bed and eating hospital food only made me more nervous about how things were going at home. Could Ellen handle him without my help? After all, doesn't the world revolve around Indispensable Bob?

But I returned to find that the family had not fallen off a cliff. Ellen had handled everything smoothly. Two-year-old Dave greeted me with a hug.

But Walker was the big surprise.

As soon as I stepped into the living room, he grabbed my hand and took me over to the couch. He picked up a Disney read-along-with-a-tape book of *Pinocchio*. Sitting beside me, he turned to the page where Pinocchio saves his father from the belly of a whale and pointed: *Read this to me*, he signaled with a finger.

I stared; Ellen stared. I was amazed, proud, and not a little ashamed. He was telling me he loved me. The concerns were not all on my side, as my tiny mind had assumed. Walker had worried about *me*. He would save me if he could. I hadn't given him credit for understanding the reason I'd gone to the hospital, despite all the concerned talk he had heard about it.

Giving him credit.

This was a huge issue; sometimes it seemed to be *the* issue. Because he was a non-converser, and because he seemed obsessed to the point of distraction so much of the time, we didn't give him credit for being a thinking, observing, evaluating, empathizing, *human* member of the household. Of course, we thought we knew all this. We were the great booster parents who were gifted at seeing the Real Boy behind autism's screen. We were the ones happy to lecture a teacher or therapist or doctor or relative about how normal he was despite his odd behavior. Hadn't we been the ones who reassured friends that despite Walker's not making eye contact at the right time or not showing appreciation for a gift, he really did love them? Hadn't we spoken for him in situations where he seemed shut off from the group?

Yet we regularly forgot all this and could be surprised at a moment like the Pinocchio Incident. This episode became a core story for us. We would have occasion to say often to each other, "Remember when Walker wanted to read about Pinocchio saving his father?" This was our reminder to ourselves that we regularly, consistently failed to *get him*: that our non-conversing son wasn't a loved pet that we were taking care of, but rather a person like us, with his own views, his own attachments, his own imaginative life. He had agendas, expectations, preferences, fears. He had *reasons* for doing whatever he was doing, no matter how mysterious his doings seemed to us.

And in the fall of 2013, when Walker was 28, we still—yet again!—had to relearn the lesson of the Pinocchio Incident.

Mary and April of the Hope Institute, the women who were doing the "crisis intervention" to help Walker, were scheduled to come over to our house to see him in his home habitat. They had already observed him at the vocational center and reported on how miserably he was doing. Emotionally shut off from the busy, loud room full of activity, Walker was truly—in the tired, misleading phrase about autistic people—"lost in a world of his own." Sitting at a table and refusing to cooperate with, even physically resisting, his job coach, or sitting at the door to the outside, taking his shoes off and putting them back on, Walker was a miserable young man. Unlike the agency staff, however, Mary and April weren't in knee-jerk fashion blaming him for his troubles. They were perfectly willing to entertain the idea that his environment was a big causal factor.

Unfortunately, Walker wasn't doing all that much better at home. He was more cooperative, to be sure, and less agitated than at the voc center or at his group home. But he was still a moment-by-moment challenge for Ellen and me. Our long walk through the city was his best moment each day, but this was no opportunity for others to observe him. Uninterested in eating his usual treats and entrees from the three basic food groups (spaghetti, popcorn, pizza), his most frequent demands were to get out of the house for "Zoo–Train–Walk" or to ride in the car to a distant destination. In the house he would occasionally watch his favorite music videos, but usually he just demanded that we write schedules for him.

Walker: I want pen.

Parent: OK, man. Let's write a schedule. Here's the pen. Here's the paper. Now what should we write first?

Walker: I want pen!

Parent: Now, Walker, don't shout "I" like that. Ask politely. What do we say?

Walker: I want pen, please!

Parent: What do you want to write first? How about watch a Clint Black video?

Walker: I want pen!

[repeat]

The day arrived for Mary and April's visit, and this was the signal for huge stress on our part. We had been contending that the young man they observed at the voc center was not the one we saw at home, that the guy they'd seen—difficult, upset, aggressive—was not the "real" one. But we knew Walker had changed. The formerly bright, charming, cooperative, and cheerful person was now nowhere in sight. We knew that his environment had created this change in him, but we had no way to "prove" this to anybody, especially to people who had never seen the "old" Walker.

If the same person they'd seen before put on a similar performance in his family home, we were in big trouble. This would now be two organizations—the agency and an outside organization, the Hope Institute—writing the same profile: he was a violent person who needed to live in some kind of physical restraint situation. Pam had already suggested to us that he would need a program that dealt exclusively with violent young adults. At this point in time, the agency had already kicked him out of his group home and voc program—he was currently only sleeping in his bedroom at the CILA.

So we prepared for their arrival in the only way we knew how. We would clear off the dining-room table and, when the doorbell rang, spring into action. I would present Walker with his favorite treat, a piece of French silk chocolate pie, and after he finished that in 45 seconds (or, quite probably, refused to eat it at all), I'd sit down next to him and try to entice him into watching a music video or two on his iPad, or try writing lists of promises of wonderful things we'd do when the visitors left. And always there was a small cooking timer in my hand.

This timer was a critical part of the regimen for controlling Walker. We had a supply of about five of these scattered around the house. When Walker was done with a treat, I would set one for, say, half an hour before he could have anything else to eat. If he pushed too hard—on some occasions, *physically* push—I would take him into the back porch room for a five-minute time out. This was a break for me just as much as for him. I would set the timer on my iPhone for five minutes, sit next to him in a chair, and make what passed for an entertaining game of counting the seconds and minutes with him and experimenting with various silly alarms for the end of time out. This sometimes worked to calm him down and sometimes didn't. But it was a brief escape from the insistent demands.

So plan A was this: while I scrambled with him at the table, setting timers and making promises, Ellen would do her lively-ambassador-to-the-outside-world routine, chatting with the two visitors and pretending things were fine in the Hughes family.

It was, all in all, a pathetic plan. There was no plan B.

But all of this calculation about our performance for the visitors left out one actual, breathing, thinking person: the young man himself.

→ ←

The dreaded doorbell rang and April and Mary, glowing and friendly, entered the house. I was sitting at the table with Walker and already pushing the piece of pie on him. Mary stepped over to him and said, "Hi, Walker."

His face lit up. The pie was history. He stood and went over to her and stood in front of her, smiling as at an old friend. Then he stood in front of April, grinning, and, if I'm not mistaken, flirty.

He sat down between them for a while on the couch, looking into their eyes and sending crush waves their way, then went over to the table again. He proceeded to watch several videos with me—you know, just a quiet guy enjoying country music with his dad. No trace of agitation. No "*I* want pen!" No "Zoo–Train–Walk!" I wrote a new list for him, but it wasn't necessary. He held it in his hand and stood up in his corner, grinning.

After talking for some minutes about the neighborhood, the house, the weather, April said quietly to us, "This is very different. I've never seen him this relaxed and happy before. It's remarkable."

You betcha it is! I thought. *Where the heck did this guy come from?*

"He knows you from the voc center. He likes you," Ellen said.

"Yes, but he never showed this kind of reaction to us when we were there."

They were getting a glimpse of the old Walker, the pre-trouble Walker, and were amazed.

So were we. This was the old Walker to be sure, but also a new socially connected fellow Ellen and I had never seen before. He was a person in the room with something at stake too. Like a job candidate, or a guy on a first date, he had turned on his best self.

What would he say about this if he could?

Dad, it's not such a big deal. I like Mary and April. They're nice. I know them from voc, but I'm always so crazy and upset there that I could never get to know them like I do other people. I listen to you guys, so I know why they were here. You and Mom have been talking about them coming over for weeks now. I've been looking forward to their visit. Also they're important people who might be able to help me. I'm very unhappy at voc and at the CILA. You and Mom say it all the time that they might be able to help me get a new house and a new voc center. Plus I just like them. They don't talk to me the way Debra and Daryl and Tammy do. They are a big chance for me. Also, as you know, I like girls!

This interview was a bright sparkling moment that we tucked firmly into our minds and discussed, in hopeful tones, over the next few weeks. It was a wonderful small thing to offset the mountain of worry.

Prominent on the mountain was this question: Where could he live? We, or rather Ellen, had begun to check group homes and vocational programs. The ones she visited had little experience with autism despite the headlines indicating that autism rates were going up sharply. The state of Illinois, its head stuck deep in the sand up to its shoulder blades on the issue of adults with disabilities, showed no awareness of the emergency.

The most promising group homes had astronomical waiting lists. Walker had an assigned social worker—one associated with his group home—who was supposed to help us find some place for him to live. She suggested that there are private homes approved by the state that might take him in. They are like group homes, she said, but are for individuals.

"You mean we would entrust our six-foot-three young man, who comes with a reputation for violence, to a stranger?!" I said to Ellen when she reported this suggestion. "Some 'family' would have a bedroom for him and 'take care' of him? Somebody who could handle him better than you and I and better than the so-called trained staff at the CILA? Is she nuts?"

"She's not nuts," Ellen said. "She's just blowing us off. She's fallen for the whole line the CILA is pitching about Walker and is just hoping we go away. They'll say any contradictory thing at this point. They just want us gone."

For us, the mere act of meeting with a person at a new agency was a problem. The two of us couldn't actually go to an interview together because one of us had to be with Walker. Pam offered to assign a staff member to be with him while we talked to people at a new place, but she made it clear that it would be a rough experience for him and for the staff. She said at one point that if Walker became too much of a problem, they would have to call the police to take him to a hospital because they couldn't risk hurting a staff member. Her subtext, of course, was that calling the police was exactly what they expected.

Another source of anxiety was his health. He was beginning to look alarmingly thin.

In the dark, cold early evenings of late November, we would pile into the car and take him for a temptation tour of the usual food franchise suspects. One visit to Burger King stands out. We had driven for a couple of hours and decided to pull into the Home of the Whopper. We bought a big proportion of the menu: cheeseburger, fries, apple pie, chocolate cookies, ice cream, and, of course, a Coke the size of a village water tower. We three sat tucked into a booth, and Walker looked down at his tray. He made a mighty effort. He picked up a French fry and ate half. He sipped a little bit of Coke. He nibbled at the cookie. All this time his parents prattled on: "Come on, man! Doesn't that cheeseburger look good? And ice cream! With chocolate sauce! That's fantastic." Unsmiling, uninterested, Walker just pushed to get back into the car. I sat across from him, churning with worry. Why was he, our former quarterback-size charmer, so gaunt and anxious and miserable?

We knew he was in big trouble. We took him to see the neurologist from his hospital stay who knew his recent medical situation. He suggested that Walker could have gastritis. He said it's rather common in bad group homes, especially for residents experiencing great stress. We immediately made an appointment with a gastroenterologist for an endoscope procedure.

For neurotypicals, putting a scope down the throat to diagnose gastritis is a breeze. It involves an anesthesiologist painlessly putting the patient under, and, in what seems a moment, the patient is awake and listening to a diagnosis. It's an outpatient procedure; for the patient (if not for the doctor), it's a piece of cake.

For the parents of Walker Hughes, there was no piece of cake about it, not at all. It was going to be a Very Big Deal. Just for starters, this was a young man who *would not* willingly sit or lie down on an examining table. His long-time doctor and object of worship, Frank Weschler, knew this well. On a typical visit, Walker sat, smiling and adoring, while the doctor twisted himself into a pretzel to examine him standing or sitting in a chair. *Want to take my blood pressure, doctor? Sure! Come on over here to my defensive chair! Want to take a blood sample, nurse? Love it! Just come over here to my chair where I'm safe. No problem!*

This routine was quite familiar to us in other contexts. When he was very young, we could walk into a friend's house and lose track of him immediately. We'd look all over the place and find him in a corner, upstairs, at the farthest point from the front door that he could find. The price of autism, like that of liberty in the famous phrase of Thomas Jefferson, is "eternal vigilance."

→ ←

The first and hardest step was doctor preparation. It was and will be forever thus unto the consummation of the world.

The problem was this: Getting a physician's secretary or nurse to understand via telephone that our son would not—

even with a gun to the head, even with the threat of never listening to a Clint Black tape again—willingly recline supinely on an examining table.

The Dentist Incident of some years before was a good example. Walker had to have a dental exam. It was a requirement of the CILA, and a good one. The dental clinic was one financed by the state of Illinois, which, in its generosity, would underwrite one dental visit a year, and appointments had to be made eight months in advance. This was a clinic especially geared for disabled people, and so we felt some confidence that they would understand the situation.

When Ellen made the original appointment, she iterated and reiterated our strange requirement. "Oh, no problem, Mrs. Hughes. We're used to everything here" was the reply. When the fateful day arrived, Ellen again called them and again reminded them. "Ha ha, Mrs. Hughes. It will be no problem for the doctor. We can give him a sedative in the waiting room."

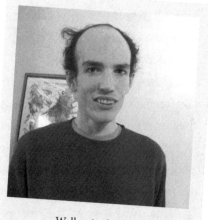

Walker in distress

"It's got to be a powerful sedative," Ellen said. "Walker can power through most pills. He thinks his life is at stake, you see."

"Oh, I know, Mrs. Hughes. We've seen everything here," the nurse chirped.

When we arrived at the clinic, located not far from our house in our densely populated, heavily trafficked Lakeview neighborhood, I double-parked so Ellen could escort Walker through the door while I hunted down a parking space. But once again we hadn't accounted for the third person in our little group. Walker would not get out of the car. Usually eager to meet doctors, normally zestfully curious about hospitals, Walker sniffed out trouble.

We coaxed. We begged. We threatened. (Or maybe we started by threatening—I don't want to remember.) He'd have none of it. We'd open the minivan door and he'd slam it shut. Ellen went in and explained the situation to the staff. Several young, eager men and women came out. A lovely female nurse with a winning manner talked to Walker and seemed to make some headway. I would have bet on this woman. But I would have lost. He was having none of this. He wanted to go home and he wanted to go *now*.

They gave him lorazepam, and we waited—to the consternation of drivers trying to get around our little street theater scene. The medication was also a no-go.

So we had to go back in a few weeks, and they gave him a shot of something stronger so he could be wheeled into the dental chair—for a mere checkup, which he passed with an A.

This was why the proposed scope-down-the-throat procedure was an all-alarm moment for the Hugheses. Ellen made the call to the specialist's nurse. Following rigid protocol, she explained in detail our conditions and got the usual response: "Ha ha. Yes, of course we'll be prepared for that. I'm afraid we've seen everything here!"

"You understand, right? It's very important. You'll have to administer some powerful sedative to Walker while he's sitting in a chair. Or maybe you can do the procedure with him right in the chair itself. I don't know. It's just that he won't get on the examining table, even for the anesthesiologist. He really won't get on an examining table at all."

"Oh, I'm sure we can handle it. The doctor will know just what to do."

These were spooky words and faint, foreboding music played in our heads, but we were determined. Walker was so sick-looking and sad that it seemed to us his life depended on a successful exam. The good news about the appointment was that it was in just two days; the bad news was that it was at two o'clock in the afternoon.

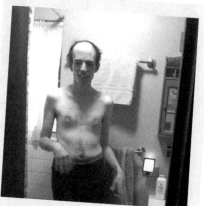

Walker, shockingly thin

This meant that Walker had to fast from the moment he got up in the morning until that time.

Now, although he was with us all day, every day, he still slept at his group home. We still wanted him to be there at night because he slept so badly at home. We thus had to impress on the staff that he could not eat anything when he got up that morning. And he could not eat anything or drink anything other than water until 2 p.m. Fortunately for the fast, he wasn't very interested in food. But he hadn't lost his appetite entirely. For him, eating and drinking were not just driven by hunger and thirst. Like anyone—but much more so than nearly everyone—his eating and drinking were part of an ironclad, never-to-be-veered-from schedule. He wouldn't consume a whole serving of fries in the condition he was in, but he would want a sip of Coke or a spoonful of ice cream or a bite of a cheeseburger. For him, the frequent possibility of food and drink was a reflex, part of the schedule of his days. Ellen and I knew this, and knew it was going to be a long, long morning.

We picked him up from the CILA, took him home, and tried to entertain him there. Already he was demanding the usual food; already we were repeating the explanation of the ban on dining. After his procedure, we promised, he could consume the planet as far as we were concerned.

At ten o'clock, with four hours to go, we decided to take him for a drive, but a drive sans treats. Our ultimate destination was the Woodfield Shopping Mall, an hour and a half away, with many stops in between. I drove. Ellen wrote. It was trouble from the start. Clutching a big stack of index cards in the back seat, Ellen wrote, "Lincolnwood Town Center Mall–gas station–Menards–forest preserve–Barnes and Noble–Woodfield Mall–doctor test." She'd read the list aloud and pass it to Walker in the front passenger seat. The trouble with this list was that it implied treats: Walker normally got a drink or cookie or roll at each stop. (The tale of how this "bad" habit developed over the years is too difficult to get into now. I can't defend it except to say, you had to be there…)

We motored nervously on Lincoln Avenue, on the expressway, on side streets. We traversed strip-mall-festooned highways and forest preserves. Inside the car we chattered and chirped and cajoled. I'd turn on the car radio hoping to distract him. "No *this* today!" he'd say as he turned it off. I was doing pretty well, performing my best Calm Father impression, as I sometimes do when I plan my emotional state ahead of time. I stoically gripped the steering wheel and stoically smiled at my anxious son all the way to Schaumburg. Of course, none of the destinations meant the usual payoff in offered treats. He'd demand ice cream and cookies and fries and root beer and he wouldn't get them.

But the situation was building.

We walked through the huge mall for a while. Over the years it became clear to us that what he loved about a mall was the *show*, the spectacle, not the consumer goods on display. Neurotypicals like me think, as they walk through a mall, *What do I want? Do I crave anything in that store? In that one?* Some places in a mall—for me, a book store or a clothing store or a sporting goods store—present me with the pleasing torment of wanting stuff. Not so for Walker. What he wants is to be with people, look at people, be in the world. You can see it in his high, happy, forward-tilting, springing walk, his head held high, a smile on his face. He's taking it all in: the bright store fronts, the little kids, the moms and dads, the young women. On the few occasions he's actually picked up a book or sweater to look at, we buy the item immediately. The only dispute has been over treats, and even those disputes are pretty fleeting.

But this day there was no high-stepping, no raised head in glowing appreciation of existence. This was, for the record, a very bad day.

After a brief unsatisfying walk through part of the mall, we got back in the car again and proceeded the same way with new lists. There were now two hours to go. After a few minutes, Ellen said, "I just can't stand it anymore. It's driving me nuts. Can I drive and you write?"

My continuing stoic self said, "Sure! It's my turn."

So I pulled off the road and we switched. This time I sat in the back seat with Walker and Ellen sat alone in the front driving.

Then Walker started a new demand: "Pepsi!" I don't know where this came from. I'm a Coke man myself and have always pushed this beverage on him, not the rival inferior drink. But I wrote: "First, we drive some more. Then we get on the expressway. Then we do doctor test. Then Pepsi." He took the card from me and shouted "Pepsi!" again. Again I wrote, and so on, and so on.

I was in the zone. I was determined to be the Michael Jordan of repeating lists. Nothing could faze me. Unfortunately, the car, normally roomy and comfortable, seemed to get smaller and smaller and more confined as the minutes crept by and "Pepsi!" was shouted in my ears. It began to feel claustrophobic, as if we were all in a U-boat in a World War II film, with depth charges exploding and the sailors looking sweaty and terrified. Ellen was completely silent and seemed to clutch the steering wheel tighter and tighter. My smile was now frozen on my face—a totally fake grimace masking my very dead stoic pose.

Somehow we reached 2 p.m. and the clinic. Walker walked in readily; apparently, he hoped relief was coming or just that he was one stage closer to Pepsi. We stepped into a little prep area with curtains. The anesthesiologist came in. "Hi, Walker," she said. "Could you get up on this table now?"

My eyes widened, my pulse accelerated. It was Ellen's turn to be stoic.

"No, he needs to be given something right here in this chair. I explained all this on the phone."

"Oh, no. We can't do it that way. It's not safe for the patient."

"But the nurse on the phone said there'd be no trouble."

"Oh, no," the anesthesiologist said. "Nobody told me anything about this. Is there some special reason?"

As Ellen went into Walker's biography and description of his autism, the doctor got visibly nervous.

"Is he dangerous?" she repeated several times, looking at him warily and stepping away as though she were surprised to be treating a pit bull instead of a human.

This is where Walker's psycho Dad came out of his shell and let it fly.

"You mean you are refusing to help him?! Can't you see what a state he's in! He's a very sick young man and needs help! And you're just blowing him off because it's not the usual way you do things? Aren't you ashamed of yourself?"

Word was getting around the clinic that something was happening.

The young, handsome, calm gastroenterologist arrived. "What's the trouble here?" he said.

Ellen, upset about the anesthesiologist, upset about Walker, and embarrassed by her husband, somehow managed to explain the situation calmly. The doctor said, "I'm sorry. We can give him specialized treatment at the hospital but we can't here. We don't have the equipment or people for it."

"That's not what we were told on the phone!" I was shouting now. "What's wrong with you people? If this were a war zone, you wouldn't refuse to help because you didn't have the staff for it. It's your responsibility. Can't you see how sick Walker is?"

"I'm sorry, Mr. Hughes. But it wouldn't be safe here."

I said some more stuff, but happily cannot remember the wording.

I took Walker by the hand and tugged him out to the car with me, while Ellen talked—calmly and reasonably—with the doctor.

She reported to me later, when I had settled down enough to be talked to, that the doctor immediately got on the phone to the hospital and set things up especially for Walker to do the procedure in a week. He was very caring and apologetic about the misunderstanding, Ellen said.

"Yeah? We'll see what their idea of being what they call 'prepared' for Walker at the hospital really is," I snarled.

→ ←

Well, we did see. When we arrived at the hospital early in the morning a week later, it was as though we'd entered the Walker Hughes Hospital Heaven of Gastritis Procedures. When we got to the prep room, there was no examining table in sight. The pediatric anesthesiologist, Dr. David Alspach, whose name will always be fixed in our memories as a superhero, greeted Walker like an old friend. He was laughing and charming and reassuring and completely in charge of the situation. Gripping a struggling Walker while he resisted in his protective chair, the doctor gave directions to the nurse for administering IV sedation while making jokes and smiling and telling the staff around him: "Remember it's not his fault!" When he was sedated, Walker was shifted to a wheelchair and thence to the table where a very friendly doctor performed the endoscopy. Afterward, when he awoke from the anesthesia, Walker sat up and started to get off the table. Ellen said, "No, stay right here for now, Walker."

A nurse said, "Oh, that's OK, Walker. Get up and walk around if you want to." We could have kissed her. All of this wonderful treatment, I guiltily realized, had been planned by the original gastroenterologist, the one I had exploded on a week earlier. As an autism father, I have a protocol about guilt, since it's such a damned relentless feature of my life: (1) Look my behavior straight in the eye and recognize how awful it was.

(2) Apologize to whomever I've offended (I wrote him a letter). (3) Resolve to reform and think of inspiring role models (for example, remember the girl on the bike). (4) *Fuggedaboutit!* It does my son no good to have a hangdog father moping about how awful he's been.

All of this excitement was just before Christmas. It turned out Walker did have gastritis and now had the right medication for it. We looked forward to a quick recovery. But we were still at a loss about what the future held. He still had to leave his CILA and still needed a new voc program, but we had no idea if there existed a place that would take him. Even if we found a good placement, we wondered if Walker would accept it.

We believed in him. We thought we knew his real nature. But we hadn't been living with him, day to day, for the last six years. We wondered: Did the staff at his CILA know something about him we didn't? Was the agency, as dreadful as they had become in our eyes, in part right? Had he changed in some basic way that would keep him from getting along in any home, in any voc training setting?

CHAPTER 12

Our Winter
of Discontent

WALKER WAS NOW RESET on a path to health, but Nurse Ratched was having none of it. Always the diagnostician who knew better than mere specialists, she emailed the neurologist just before the Christmas break with her medical and behavioral findings. The doctor, without answering her, forwarded her message to us. "I think I know what she's up to here, and I don't like it," he said.

> To [Walker's neurologist]:
>
> We are very concerned about Walker's behaviors...excessive OCD, getting naked, hiding in closet, getting in a female resident's bed naked, not eating, absconding into traffic, rough with staff...staffing is 2/1 because of danger to staff and self, refusing to go pretty much anywhere unless it is with parents.
>
> We would like him to be psych admitted for these excessive behaviors on Friday (?). I would request that his parents only visit for an hour or two daily because you will

not get a clear picture of his behaviors when they are there constantly. I will mention this to his mom. I think this is in his best interest. We are very very concerned about Walker.

Thanks, [Nurse Ratched]

The doctor explained that he'd seen this before. Some group homes are understaffed at Christmas time, and they use the hospital psych ward as a stopgap way to handle their clients. In addition, the Ripper-like young man she described didn't fit the mild, cooperative fellow he knew at the hospital. Here was the nurse telling him yet again that he was being fooled by these Hugheses, that their kid was a threat to civil society, and that they were trying to paper over their problem by manipulating him. He said he would refuse to admit Walker yet again into the psychiatric unit.

The accusations she was making were hateful and bizarre. She seemed to be throwing wild stories at the wall, hoping something—anything—would stick in order to get the doctor to take him off her hands. We knew that Walker's idea of a sexual "move" was to offer his cheek to a woman, as though deigning to be kissed. This portrait of a naked would-be rapist was bad sensation fiction. (We later discovered that in all the many, many pages maintained by the staff detailing Walker's misdeeds, there was no record of any "getting into a female resident's bed naked.")

So, at Christmas time, Walker's favorite time of the year, a season of family parties and music and little precious memories and traditions, the CILA nurse wanted him separated from his parents and everyone else he knew and placed in a mental ward.

Ellen and I were furious, almost literally hopping mad. Dave became alarmed and wondered what the fuss was about.

After we explained about the nurse, he dashed off one of his therapeutic cartoons to calm his parents down. All of his life, Dave had told stories about silly, goofy characters he made up. Their "problems" were always of their own making and small beyond belief, daffy parodies of real human problems. The cast had evolved over the years but the current one involved Sauce Hoss, Weezy, Fred and Fred-Fred, Dr. Spanko, Ebafleezer Hatbasket, Banjo-Bits Tompkins, and many more. He texted or emailed their opinions and comments and adventures to Ellen and me (but mainly to Ellen) every day. Sometimes they appeared on comic blogs he created with pictures. But their concerns were so off-the-wall, so blazingly bonkers in every way, that they had a soothing effect on both of us.

Dave decided it was time for the Sauce Hoss to make a rare real-life appearance, to console his parents about Nurse Ratched, so he dashed the one shown here on to one of Walker's index cards.

Dave's cartoon: The Sauce Hoss

Our dilemma was that we wanted to take him home, get him the hell away from his hostile group home, but two things blocked us: (1) We were afraid that if he lost all connection to the home, he would lose his funding from the state and no longer be able to get into any home. (2) We thought he couldn't sleep well at home and that, as a result, we wouldn't sleep either and wouldn't be able to function at work. The result was that we made sure to minimize his contact with the place, to have him all day and through the evening and drop him off late-ish, around 9 p.m., and pick him up early in the morning. This arrangement was doomed, we knew, but we wanted to prolong it at least until there was some hope for another group home on the horizon.

→→ ←←

Fortunately, the nurse backed off her threatened incarceration of Walker, and so we were able to muddle—sometimes stagger—through the Christmas holidays with him at home, day and evening. We tried and even occasionally succeeded in having the sort of Christmas we were accustomed to. He was still frighteningly thin and not especially interested in food, but he was there, with us in the house, for the tree, the cookies, the cozy fire, the music he loved. He was agitated, distracted, and pretty much unsmiling, but he was with his family, with people who liked him. The sad saga continued, however: moment by moment, he was a challenge. *How can we entertain him? How can we keep him occupied and help him relax? How can we keep our patience?* Tedious time outs with the timer in the back room were a regular feature of life.

Dave, who normally spent most of his day in the Loop on the DePaul campus with friends, was home now all day and in his room with his noise-canceling headset on. He was, happily for him, off in his own creative world, writing an extra screenplay during his "break" from screenwriting classes (he was now in the Master of Fine Arts program at DePaul) and pumping out fictions from his delightfully creative mind, just because he had to. But noise-canceling headphones go only so far to muffle trouble right outside a bedroom door. Sometimes he just set off—in the sub-zero cold of those days—to walk, to go to a library to work, even to take a long train ride to a far suburb to be somewhere else. His parents were no longer as available for normal chit-chat as they had been when Walker was busy during the week.

→ ←

After the holidays, life returned to the current normal. I began teaching a class part-time at my college and Dave returned to his classes at DePaul. The agency in its generosity had agreed to take care of Walker on Tuesday and Thursday mornings while I taught and Ellen tried to get some work done. But this routine only lasted until the fateful day, January 22nd, when we effectively cut all ties with the agency and Walker came home to live 24/7.

The first few days that Walker was home were a time of critical, heart-thumping anxiety for us. A very good sign of the pitch that our nerves had reached was the fact that, after he had been sleeping at home for only three nights, I suddenly began writing a journal. Now I am *not* a Journal Guy. I don't have the energy, the get-up-and-go, to record my own daily activities. But as a Freshman Composition teacher, of course, I recommend journal or diary writing all the time. I tell my students how it helps them lead the Socratic Examined Life and that they will be fascinated to read the journal years from now when they have forgotten the mental place they were in at this moment. I tell them that their children and grandchildren will get a kick out of reading old Grandma and Grandpa's diaries 50 years from now and that it will be a fine historical record of How People Lived Back in the Day. I tell them about one of my favorite books, *The Diary of Samuel Pepys*, and how valuable his unpretentious, starkly honest, and diligently kept entries have been to readers for hundreds of years.

But it was all hypocritical (if sincerely meant!) gassing from their old baby-boomer teacher. Until this moment in January 2014, I'd never written a single sentence of a journal. However, the times were exceptional enough even for me, as Walker says, to "Write Stuff Down." A couple of things to notice: (1) The volume here is a couple of decibels higher than the rest of this book, showing how exceptional the times really were for us. (2) It's just a fragment, ending about a week after it started, showing how lazy the writer really is.

⇝ ⇜ ⇝ ⇜

Saturday, January 25, 2014, 8:45 p.m. The impossible is happening right now: Walker is upstairs lying down quietly, Ellen is typing on her laptop. I'm typing on this laptop. Walker isn't shouting, isn't trying to push an agenda into next week, next year. The TV is off. Peace reigns. But this isn't 1986 or 1992 or 1997. This is NOW, the worst, most prolonged spell of Walker Anxiety we have ever experienced.

On Thursday, I came home from my morning class and sat down for a moment with Ellen on the couch before getting in the car to pick up Walker at the group home and give him a break from his prison-hell existence for a 6-hour reprieve of a walk and/or drive and some eating to try to boost his emaciated frame. E was about to go to FF [her employer for her part-time grant-writing job] and try to make a stab at increasing her freelancing. Then Pam calls and tells Ellen that W has been wild and uncontrollable and tried to choke a staff member and MUST go the psych ward (AGAIN!), for the 3rd time in what? 4 months. E just listens, doesn't say a word, and says we'll pick him up and call the neurologist.

We pick up our young Madman and staff strangler and he's all smiles, all friendliness. We drive to say hi to Grandma Ruth [my mother, who lived an hour and a half away in Schaumburg] and plot our next move. E calls the neurologist and he says there's no bed available but maybe tomorrow. So we decide to keep him home that night and brace ourselves for the worst. For months W has been a moment-by-moment challenge. Always pushing, shouting for the next active thing on his list and never, ever relaxing. He's gotten less verbal and more pushy and won't read my notes. We assume he won't sleep so we bought earplugs.

But he's happy at home, even relaxed. We're amazed and relieved but tense. When will the shouting start? The minutes tick by and no trouble. HOW CAN THIS BE? He sleeps on the mattress on the living-room floor very soundly. He gets up at 5 but remains quiet and does not, as I feared he would, run up and down the stairs to tug on us to get up and get going, going.

We eventually rise and make a big breakfast and he eats it ravenously. All the time he's quiet and smiling. I read the paper. No, you're not hallucinating, Bob. I read the paper. Slowly and uninterruptedly. He's so quiet and cooperative we begin to realize a change of plan: we don't want him to go to no psych ward and the doctor won't want it either. I decide to drive to Gurnee, download a new audiobook, and we set out. E stays home and calls the neurologist. He has a theory (a theory I voiced the night before, I had it first!) that agency people have provoked him and/or they are simply lying about the choking. (They have repeatedly accused him of slapping and punching and endangering human life; we have never believed it and never see it at home, and he's been home A LOT lately.) That they want to put him in the psych ward and will refuse to take him back when he gets out. Our great friend and snake Pam calls again to "see how we're doing." E lets her have it, albeit calmly, and tells her we know what they're up to.

The rest of the day, this is Friday now, goes by in a haze of peace, happiness, relaxed cooperative behavior from W and TOTAL AMAZEMENT. WTF!? We had not seen this kind of happiness on his face or relaxation in years. He steps into the house after our drive and wants to see "The Muppet Christmas Carol"!! He wouldn't even watch it a couple of weeks ago. He wants to listen to music. He actually exists in the house without pushing his hysterical OCD agenda, nailing down the sequence of future existence to keep it from vaporizing.

This is the biggest change we've seen in him in months, years even. The only approach to this was in the psych ward, where he relaxed a bit from his prison sentence and watched "Old School," but he was nothing like this happy there.

That night he slept well again, was quiet in the morning AGAIN, and AGAIN did not do his running-up-and-down-the-stairs-to-get-us-up routine—the routine I feared the most. NONE of our fears about having him in the house have materialized.

Today I drove him to Gurnee again, he ate like a trencherman, we had a happy extra long walk in 16-degree weather (my knees are miraculously doing better and he is stronger now).

It's now 9:18 p.m. and he's still happy, laughing, and quiet. E and I both swear he will never sleep in that CILA again. We'll meet with Clearbrook [an agency that looked promising] people this week and move as fast as we can. W, thank God and thank

W himself, is way more presentable now than we feared he would be when they took a look at him.

Just took a little video of Walker delightedly playing air guitar to a Clint Black song with Ellen.

→ ←

Tuesday, January 28, 2014, 7:08 p.m. Walker was pleased with our usual routine of Gurnee drive then ZTW. He's becoming more agitated as his lack of activity and firm schedule wears on. But he's happy and talks a little bit, sometimes surprisingly. When he got home tired from our walk in 2-below weather today at 5 and we asked him if he wanted pizza, he said "Later." Later?!!!

Ellen had a very unsettling email exchange with Pam yesterday. First a phone call in which E asked if the CILA people could watch Walker a couple of times when we meet with other agencies to try to find a new placement and Pam responding that sure they will, but they expect to have to call the fire dept. or police and have him taken to the hospital because he's so violent. Ellen said nothing in response but waited and wrote this email:

> From: Ellen Hughes
> To: [Pam]
> Date: Mon, Jan 27, 2014 at 3:14 PM
> Subject: To be clear
>
> Recapping your phone call to me an hour ago:
>
> In response to our request for the Agency's help in caring for Walker during important upcoming meetings with other agencies now that we are caring for Walker at home full-time, you called to warn me that you fully anticipate

that Walker will be violent right away at the CILA, a great danger to your staff and himself, and you will immediately call for emergency personnel—fire dept, police—to transport him first to an emergency room at a local hospital, and from there to the [hospital] psych ward.

You wanted to be very sure I understood that rather than help us and help Walker make this difficult transition away from the Agency, you and your staff intend to immediately call emergency services to remove him from your care.

The facts here:

» Walker has been at the CILA for six years and has known you for much longer, he's a guy you know very well, who thinks you are his friend.

» You have a team of skilled autism professionals there, but you would immediately turn this scared guy over to emergency squad personnel, police officers, ER staff.

» You don't have any idea how to entertain Walker for a couple hours peacefully. No idea at all. So you can't and won't help us.

» Walker still technically resides at the CILA and is funded for a one-on-one aide.

In this difficult situation, you thought only of how to distance yourself from Walker's distress. You have spent NO time thinking how you could use the resources you have to help him. You are thinking only of distancing yourself from him.

Robert and I are just amazed.

Ellen

→ ←

This morning I was getting more and more anxious about how W can be handled when I go to school this Thursday. E trying to mollify me and reassure me. I have so much trouble with not knowing how things will go in the near future, always I do. But I'm very glad W is stronger and happier. Call my mood Anxious Happiness or Happy Anxiety.

Despite the extreme cold, W was a very enthusiastic trekker today. Absolutely nobody was out, but WE were, happy Antarctic explorers. I was proud of his attitude. The weather has been monstrously cold, the high below zero. Hard to stay out very long.

Wednesday, January 29, 2014, 8:24 a.m. Just a note: I'm trying to eat breakfast and read the paper, but W is shouting for the last hour "ride in car." This is in sharp contrast to last Friday, the first morning, when we read the paper at leisure while he smilingly waited. He's getting more anxious, with good reason. So are we. BUT, once again last night, as every night so far in this new 24/7 Walker-on-board existence, we had a very good, uninterrupted, sound sleep. The sleep itself is a big surprise and continues to be.

Thursday, January 30, 2014, 8:49 p.m. This is the one-week mark—he's been home for a week and the pressure of his uncertain life is starting to show. He was pretty unsettled today. E and D drove him around while I was at school and all went well. He was pretty rattled and OCDish on our walk (which did last a long 2.5 hours, but with a lot of shouted repeated wishes). This evening has been our first troubled one. Instead of going upstairs and resting quietly while we read, he's been hassling us about getting "SQUARE PIE" without any letup. No matter how much we spell out exactly how we'll buy one for tomorrow, he won't acknowledge that he understands (or believes?) it. He just hammers away at it. This minute he's trying to get E and me to go to bed and turn off all lights. He wants the whole house to conform to his every wish. Rough stuff.

⇥ ⇤

Friday, January 31, 2014, 9:20 p.m. OK, simply the most AMAZING day:

It started badly, with W getting up in the same shouty, anxious mood he went to sleep in (though he did sleep well). He simply perseverated on The Next Thing all day, shouting, being inaccessible, even rather hostile. E and I drove with him to IKEA, him shouting all the way in the back seat, repeating "IKEA!" or some other word. Can't remember. By the time we returned to Chicago and got in line at Jewel, he was driving us nuts, constantly making an "AHHH Ahhhh Ahhh" noise loudly. At home it got worse and worse and we called the neurologist. We even filmed him to show how overwhelming he was.

He had been home one week. Had been good the first 4 days, but for the last two was becoming more anxious, hitting a peak this afternoon.

We assumed the doc would want him in the psych ward. Instead he doubled W's Geodon [a drug that helps control behavior]. E gave it to him right away, I gave him a shower and we went for a ZTW, successfully. At home again he was cooperative, peaceful, ate a lot, watched videos with E, watched

"Talledega Nights" about a third of the way through and THE ENTIRE MOVIE "OLD SCHOOL"!!! All the time, no "AHHH AHHH AHH," no shouting, no pushing, just cooperative and wanting to do real things, like watch videos and movies. Hurray, Geodon.

We've never witnessed such a transformation, such a Hyde to Jeckyll day. And it absolutely was the Geodon, nothing E and I did. He's behaving right now the way he did at UIC hospital: showing the kind of cooperative, nice guy he really is. We were getting very very alarmed today about Clearbrook coming over in one week to look at him and seeing a wild uncontrollable guy. We feel much relieved and much less anxious about that (as of now, 9:23 p.m.).

This minute he's sitting with E and thinking of song titles for her to find on YouTube. He's thinking and enunciating and peaceful. Oh my.

⟶ ⟵

Sunday, February 2, 2014, 8:55 a.m. Well, yesterday, like the day before was "go 100 m.p.h. in one direction, hit reverse, go 100 m.p.h. in the other direction."

It was Saturday, the morning after the Great Happiness Evening, and E, W, and I were getting in the car. E was going to Bernice's for coffee. Snowing heavily. Then Walker's tongue swelled like a balloon and his speech became very slurred. So on to Evanston Hospital, fast, as his symptoms get worse. In the ER the staff was very professional, swift, kind, smart. It could be a reaction to the Geodon, which had been doubled the day before. Or to his BP med or eggs or...

W good all day in the ER first, then in "observation," which entails almost no observations. Beautiful Evanston snowfall out the window. W planted in place, behaving very well, very still really and very cooperative. BUT the two of us ready for uncontrollable explosions which never happened. Exhausting.

Went home at 6 p.m. with very bad result: no Geodon, the doctors say, it could be the problem, and give him prednisone, which (sorry!) will make him agitated. At home, we got agitation all right, him revving up up up. Our worry through the roof. And, of course, what about his alarm at himself and pain? E emails the neurologist who calls back. He says they're all wrong, no allergy, just a dystonic reaction to Geodon. Give him Benadryl and it will clear up right away. So this morning we face the day with a calmer guy, cooperative, and I am looking forward to long ride with him while I listen to a new book (please be good!)—"Into Africa" about Stanley and Livingston. It's part of my Victorian expedition kick. I loved "Endurance" by Alfred Lansing.

→ ←

Thursday, February 6, 2014, 5:52 p.m. So, last Tues, the 4th, was amazing. Ellen woke up with a very very bad neck, I had to teach class, and E had a meeting re more freelancing. Our prediction: disaster, because through it all we had to handle Walkman. Surprise! He stayed upstairs all day lying in, coming down to eat, being pleasant. Everything worked out. How do you spell relief?

Wed. was good. Had a 3-hr walk in the cold with him, came home and watched all of "Talledega Nights." Gag "Walker Texas Ranger" gets me every time. Again, go figure. He seems to be relaxing.

I taught today, Thurs, E took W to IKEA in the morning and all worked out well. At one point E asked him, "Is that what you want?" He answers, "It's what I want." Note: "It's"?!!!!! A pronoun! Not repetition! Holy shit. Conversationalese emerges now and then, when he's relaxed and doesn't seem self-conscious. He's also, annoyingly, saying "Ahhhhh" almost all day today, no letup. Is it self-comforting, because he's rattled? Is it related to the conversationalese that slips out? Is he trying to talk, in a way, trying to push it out? We don't know.

Had a bad walk with him. It was 2 degrees, wind chill 15 below, but he did not want to get on the bus when the icy wind was blowing in our faces. Managed to get on bus, but wanted to get off at every stop thinking we would miss riding the elevator at the Century [this is a mall and a mandatory stop on warmer days]. I didn't want to make a scene in the crowded bus, so quietly went along each time. I got pretty damn annoyed. Knees really hurt.

Right now, he's sitting with E watching Toby Keith videos. Interesting: lately he's been saying "Obama." So we turn on the news. That's not it. Then we tried watching a video of the State of the Union speech. He loved it. Mesmerized watching Obama for about 10 minutes. Very strange. Very good.

By the way, every single night he's been home, he has slept well. This was our biggest fear of all, that we wouldn't get any sleep. It's been a very good thing.

→ ← → ←

Re-reading this meager attempt at a "journal," I'm struck by a few features. One is how eager we were to hear Walker talk—not just enunciate words but say things that approximate what we think of as "comments." When he was first in the CILA, his speech picked up. Under the positive influence of Doug and Caroline, he made some strides forward. But in the last couple of years, since the CILA became a sort of holding facility, he had become much more silent. The few new words he came out with in his first week home with us were thus momentous. They signaled a healthy change.

All his life we have looked at our normal—pardon me, better-than-normal-looking son—and dearly, desperately wanted to know his thoughts. Any little comments that he made, sometimes very surprising comments, have always been tantalizing hints of the thinking soul behind autism's wall. So this new guy, intermittently relaxed enough to think out loud, was a revelation.

Another striking thing here is the shocking break from Ellen's philosophy of diplomacy. Her idea, adhered to under extremely trying circumstances, was to smile and be polite and encouraging to the staff, even when provoked. Her policy may even have been over-compensation for her husband's touchy personality. She always said (and I've always agreed—in theory anyway) that you can yell righteously at people and get the result you want just once—only once. After that, they see you coming and they run the other way. They don't answer your calls. They don't respond to emails. You need to treat people as if they are trying to do good and as if you are trying to aid them in their attempt. Her email message here was the last straw, an outpouring after all the civil conversational bridges had been burned.

And the panic that comes through here. Walker was recovering, yes, but could he recover enough to "behave" the way he would be expected to at a new group home and a new voc program? Maybe he wanted to live with us. Maybe he was sick of the whole group home and voc ed world. Maybe he was only calm (and then only relative to agency life) when he was with us. But good luck with that, we thought, since we parents would not always be around. Finding a good group home was one thing, a very iffy thing. But would he balk at *any* new living arrangement?

We just couldn't know.

CHAPTER 13

Hold On, Partner

IF A PICTURE IS worth a thousand words, a brief video must be worth—what?—2500 words? This equation is the iPhone generation's philosophy of journaling and it became ours too, in a way. As I lost ambition and quit writing my so-called diary, I stepped up the moving- and still-picture taking. There were two reasons for this: (1) When any sign of the old, happy, connected Walker appeared, we wanted a record of it to remind ourselves, and possibly the staff at a new agency, that there really was a promising young man behind the obvious trouble. (2) When he seemed to be going off the rails with anxiety, we wanted something to show his doctors—behavior-modifying medications require a good look at the behavior.

A video of the first kind became a huge favorite with us, viewed again and again. On a frigid January evening, Walker shouted, "*I want ice cream!*" Ellen got him some, with Hershey's chocolate sauce and Reddi-wip, as was his wont. This continued the new eating regime: any demand for a specific item from the starving son meant he got what he wanted. He promptly ate the whipped cream and chocolate sauce, ignored the ice cream, stood up, and started a new refrain: "*I want popcorn party!*"

"No, Walker. You've got to finish your ice cream before you have popcorn," Ellen told him, proving that we do have gastronomic standards in the family.

"Popcorn party! Popcorn party!" he repeated, this time approaching Ellen and getting a little pushy. He stepped close to her with a pen and index card in his hand. "Popcorn party! Write stuff down!" he said. This was a bad sign, one that these days meant he might grab her and that I'd be taking him into the back room for a time out.

"Let's sit down and write," Ellen said. So they sat together on the couch. I watched all this from My Chair in the corner of our living room. Sometimes I wisely opted out of trouble because my intervention just served to raise the temperature of the room.

The protocol demanded that Ellen write a brief list, a sequence, that Walker could read and absorb and help him to calm down, such as "Finish ice cream—Wait 20 minutes—Then popcorn party." He'd hold the card and timer in his hands and refer to them in an agitated way as he danced a few steps forward, then a few steps backward in his station in the dining area.

Ellen decided to live on the wild side and break with protocol. She wrote, "Only a lunatic would ask for popcorn while his ice cream is melting on the table." Walker read this quietly to himself and burst out laughing. Then he gave it back to her and, still laughing, said, "Popcorn!" Ellen pointed to the card again. Then the laughter gripped him and would not let him go.

I picked up my phone and turned it on. The video shows him giggling uncontrollably as Ellen rewrote the sentence again and again. Each time he read it aloud and—skinny shoulders shaking, eyes filling with tears, and mouth wide open in convulsive laughter—he'd lean over to Ellen's face and stare into her eyes as if he couldn't believe his mom was such an amazing comedian.

Everything was there in a one-minute video: his intelligence, his un-autistic sense of irony, his loving nature, his good cheer, his charm. Thank you, Apple, Inc.

→ ←

Another video of the first kind could be called "The Young Air Guitarist." He's sitting close to Ellen on the couch and listening to "A Good Run of Bad Luck," a Clint Black song, on YouTube. He wears a smile of total delight and is air-guitaring to beat the band. His lifelong so-called "perseverative" movement had been right arm bent at a 90-degree angle, forearm up, and left arm straight and pointed downward at a 45-degree angle, both pumping up and down. He was so continually kinetic that even still photos caught the move. In photo after photo, he smiles at the camera with his right arm raised and left arm downward in a modified semaphore letter Y or S, his right hand a blur. But by this time, in January of 2014, this signature move of his had morphed into a definite air-guitar performance. In still photos, his right hand was still a blur.

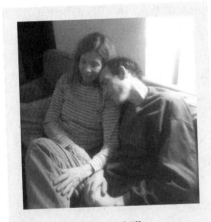
Walker and Ellen

Now his right hand strummed invisible strings and his left hand moved fast to form fantastic chords. He could air-guitar in any mood—happy, sad, even panicked. We loved it. It was as if his favorite country singers were being invisibly invoked as companions or witnesses to his daily life. Or perhaps the music itself was comforting in exactly the same way it is for the millions of music-obsessed ear-bud fetishists all around the world.

Clint Black is singing, "I'd bet it all on a good run of bad luck / Seven come eleven and she could be mine / Luck be a lady, and I'm gonna find love / comin' on the bottom line." Ellen is holding the iPad while Walker grins widely, strums his invisible strings to match the beat of the song, and works the end of the guitar neck expertly with his left hand. In the classic move of the global air-guitar community, he leans forward and sits straight up as if imagining he's Clint himself performing the song. Then he leans back on the couch and tilts his head in toward Ellen, touching his forehead to hers and gazing into her eyes. At 28, Walker still shares this loving joke with his mother. When he was a baby, Ellen would say "Bonkers!" and they'd touch foreheads and grin.

Music had been important to Walker all his life. His earliest love had been Fred Astaire and the Gershwin and Cole Porter and Irving Berlin songs we played for him. We recorded the film *Blue Skies* and would show him Fred dancing to "Puttin' on the Ritz." As a toddler, he'd play and replay this dance as if it were a music video, and he'd stare at Fred's feet and try to imitate him in front of the TV set. I used to sing many of the old songs to him while bathing him in the bathtub—"Cheek to Cheek," "Night and Day," "Isn't This a Lovely Day?"—and he'd sing along with me. He knew a very large number of songs by heart. I could stop singing anywhere in any song, and he'd continue the line for me. Singing certainly seemed to be registering in a part of his brain where relaxation and joy reigned. A boy normally paralyzed when invited to speak, who couldn't or wouldn't say "My stomach hurts," could sing the tricky, complicated lyrics to "Puttin' on the Ritz" and rattle off perfectly "The Twelve Days of Christmas."

As he got older and his parents played a country music station in the car, he became a huge fan of some singers. At the top of his list was Clint Black. At age 11, Walker had dressed like him for Halloween—black cowboy hat, black shirt, black pants. He knew every word to every hit and played the songs endlessly on his Walkman. In the psych ward, Toby Keith was the role model: his videos portrayed a world the 28-year-old Walker clearly wished he could join—single guys and girls partying. At home, he returned to his original man crush, Clint Black, whose songs are more thoughtful and musically sophisticated and, perhaps, reminded him of better times when he was a kid.

Happy videos of this first kind—"Air Guitarist" and "Only a Lunatic"—were reassuring and we checked in on them with frequent viewings.

→ ⟵

Videos of the second kind, however, were very troubling and not the stuff for repeated looks. In one taken in February, he's shouting "Zoo–Train–Walk!" over and over and shaking his right hand up and down in a modified, strenuous, and somewhat alarming air-guitar movement. In this brief video, he is standing over Ellen, who is sitting down. He's yelling "Zoo–Train–Walk" very loudly. He's hit a volume that signals he's going to get physically threatening and so Ellen is playing the whole thing down.

We learned the hard way over the years—that is, through trial and error—what the best teachers and therapists for autistic people have always known: that when a scared or very troubled autistic person gets aggressive, that is the very moment to step the mood down dramatically. You never, ever take the bait. Ellen is speaking to him casually and quietly, masking her alarm with all her might: "OK, first you have to eat your sandwich. Then you can do Zoo–Train–Walk." He's strumming faster and faster and circling around her chair, looking down at her and over at me, the goofball videographer strangely pointing an iPhone at him. The dialogue—shouting and quiet replies—repeats several times.

He keeps strumming his invisible guitar and gamely tries to comply. He backs up, going "Ah ah ah," and sits down at the table and takes a bite. With food still in his mouth, he gets up and walks over to Ellen again. This time she crosses the room to step away from him and he follows her. Sitting on a stool now with her arms folded, she says quietly, "You need to calm down. You need to take it easy." That video ends and the next one, from a few moments later, is more dire. This time Ellen is backing up down the hallway with Walker approaching her, still yelling for "Zoo–Train–Walk." He's threatening to grab her but at the last minute always backs away and looks frantically at me. We start talking over the trouble right there, about how we'll call the doctor. The two of us are acting calm, but that's all it is: an act. We're very scared and uncertain.

And guilty. It seemed to us that many of his symptoms suggested some kind of post-traumatic stress disorder: his heightened anxiety, his hypervigilance and irritability, his intense emotions, his difficulty in falling asleep and concentrating, his jumpiness. We were confident about inferring the threat of violence that he lived with at the CILA: his regular bruising from the blows of Tracey and Brandon and his reluctance to eat with the others. He had lived in a trauma-rich environment. This, coupled with the hostility of the staff, would be enough to make his life a daily nerve-wracking gauntlet. Ellen and I couldn't stand the stress of his infamous birthday party years ago. What had it been like for him to live with that birthday party for more than two years? How could we have permitted this situation to last for so long?

Compounding the trouble at the group home was Todd, the sad housemate, who surely increased Walker's stress with the depression he radiated every minute. What was it like for hypersensitive Walker to live with him? (Of course, the other question—What was life like for Todd himself?—was just as powerful an indictment of the place. How were his needs being met? How were Brandon's and Tracey's, for that matter? All were entitled to appropriate care; none was getting it.) Todd's life there was a shame, of course. Even Pam, in her honest moments, admitted that. But the bottom line was that Todd was easier than Walker and required less staffing—he could be ignored for hours. And the agency received just as much funding for Todd as it did for Walker.

Walker's hypersensitivity had always been a feature of life for us. An incident in his childhood stood out. I don't know when it was—anywhere from age six to 11. Dave and Walker were in the back seat of the car. Dave, the talking son, was demanding that we stop at McDonald's. He repeated his request over and over until we wanted to, in Ellen's signature phrase, "pull our heads off and bowl with them." Every time he asked, we said, or perhaps yelled, "No. Not now." But he wouldn't let it go. He went on and on with it, tirelessly, relentlessly. Suddenly, the non-talking son spoke up. In an agonized, frustrated voice, Walker shouted, "Say yes!" We spun around in the front seat to look at him. Even Dave was speechless for a moment. All we could think was *What the hell?*

Often Ellen and I wondered about that moment and imagined what it would be like to go through life without being able to make little statements like that, without being able to inject your own will in a normal fashion into quite humdrum situations. Even more, what would it be like to, as it were, have a sock in your mouth when emotions are high, to be unable to express yourself in a charged atmosphere? And finally, imagine living like Walker did in a group home where emotions were always high, where trouble was always around the corner, where deep depression was constantly visible.

The wonder was not that he was agitated; the wonder was that he could ever smile at all.

→ ←

Meanwhile, our nerve-wracking quest for a decent placement for Walker continued. Ellen and I, but usually Ellen alone, visited several places and talked to kindly staff persons. Most programs seemed inappropriate for Walker in one way or another, partly because autism—despite the high profile it had in the media—was not a top priority for adults. One problem was the difficulty of classifying Walker:

Kindly Staff Person: Is he intelligent?

Ellen: Yes.

KSP: Is he verbal?

Ellen: No, not in the "conversation" sense. But he does talk a little.

KSP: Can he tell you what he wants some other way, like typing on a computer?

Ellen: No.

KSP: Does he comment on things?

Ellen: No.

KSP: Is he aggressive?

Ellen: No, but… No, we don't think so, but yes, he was kicked out of his group home because he was unmanageable. We think they were incompetent, though.

KSP: I don't understand. Could you explain that?

Ellen: How much time do you have?

Another problem—a huge and gnawing one—was that we just didn't know how Walker would do in any new placement. Even at home, even with his loving and encouraging parents, he could get physically threatening, lose control, and need a time out. He required constant attention, thoughtful and alert companionship, every moment he was awake. There was no possibility, for example, that alone with him in the house I could do anything else but attend to him: play videos, read to and with him, dole out entrees and treats at precisely timed intervals, watch a film (though "watching" doesn't adequately suggest how active my participation was expected to be). Oh, and give him time outs. "Zoo–Train–Walk"—through the cold and snow—was at this time the only sure-fire pleasurable thing we both did. Even with the gastritis pain in his gut, he still craved getting out and moving. Yet every day I seriously questioned if my knees would tolerate it.

We knew that the "old Walker" was quite capable of living and working in a group home and vocational education setting. He'd done it for four years. But the turmoil of the last two years had created a different, damaged young man. Could he live somewhere new and convince people who'd never known the "old Walker" that a "better" guy was really there? Parents can put on a show and give all the testimonials they please, but when the young man shows up in all his reality, their words mean nothing.

We had talked to people at one agency that looked very good, called Clearbrook. It was big, even vast by the standards of Walker's previous placement. It had 43 group homes, most of which were in the northwest suburbs of Chicago. They too did not have a large autism program, but they were actively expanding into that area. Walker, they said, might fit the mix they planned for a new vocational ed site they were just beginning to set up in Evanston. They were very friendly and even took us to see one of their group homes.

The house was too good to be true. Each resident had his own bedroom and the common area was very homey. It was in a quiet old suburb with huge trees. To me it seemed a setting right out of a Washington Irving story—Ichabod Crane might saunter down the street any minute. Walker's former CILA, by contrast, was in a rough area of Chicago. On one occasion, his beloved friends, staffers Tony and Caroline, were chatting in front of the house when a passerby shot another guy on the sidewalk just yards from them. Ambulances perpetually pulled up to another group home for adults across the street. But even in this Dodge City locale, Walker's housemates, two of whom Ellen and I regarded as too dangerous to be near our son, were considered by the staff to be *less* dangerous than Walker.

We could only wonder, *Is Walker ready for Sleepy Hollow? Will he simply be kicked out the first day?*

A few weeks later, we visited their Evanston vocational program. They called it "CHOICE." The governing idea there was that each morning the clients could choose what they wanted to do. For example, they could choose to work with the Meals on Wheels truck, delivering food to shut-ins—disabled and elderly people who couldn't get out to grocery stores. They could opt to go to a book store, or do volunteer work on a farm, or do yoga, or make sandwiches for a foundation, engage in group games, take a walk, or go on a field trip. When Ellen and I walked in, friendly young people greeted us. We thought, *The staff certainly is nice.* Then we learned they weren't staff; they were actual clients. They showed us a semicircular table where the group met each morning and discussed their day. The rooms were quiet; no one was raising his voice. They had lessons here too and showed small educational videos and played games on a huge Smart Board.

Well, this is very civilized, we thought. Certainly Ellen and I could fit in here. Maybe we could benefit from a program like this. But Walker? The voc program at the agency found him off-the-charts wild—absolutely a loss. They thought he needed some kind of rigid policing, some highly disciplined reform-school-type structured environment.

Could Walker actually sit at their semicircular table? Could he focus long enough on any activity? Could he be friendly and gentle? Could he be quiet and—most important—stay put? We knew he was far, far less verbal than some of the clients we met. We knew his agitation level could require a physically fit intervention team. Would he be kicked out of here on the first day he arrived?

→ ←

But this season of trauma and doubt and fright about the future was momentarily obliterated by one brief moment that put everything into perspective for us. The moment was entirely engineered by Ellen, the family ambassador to the outside world. I fully admit this fact. Without her, these few minutes of euphoria never would have occurred. But it was also a moment that was redeemed by me, the Hero of the Day.

"Hero of the Day" status was one that shifted regularly around the family. The term came from the *Curious George* books that were a short-lived fad in the house when the boys were very young. Every story in the series ended with the Man in the Yellow Hat announcing that George the mayhem-causing monkey was the "Hero of the Day." We always read these words loudly and slowly and pompously, like a proclamation. For years afterward, the term became one we'd bestow on each other, or on Walker himself or on Dave, after one of us did something helpful. Sometimes, of course, the term was heavy sarcasm, but usually it was meant as a sincere, if mock-inflated, compliment.

My heroism here, though, required no false inflation.

One day, during one of our constant car trips to the suburbs, Ellen pointed silently to a sign outside the North Shore Center for the Performing Arts in Skokie. I looked but couldn't believe my eyes. It announced that in a few weeks Clint Black would be appearing there in concert. The words just appeared there, in normal-size lettering and with no special fanfare as though the

North Shore Center for the Performing Arts thought it was just another announcement and not something that might cause regular six-car pileups. *Clint Black?!* Ellen and I looked at each other, wide-eyed. *Himself? Not a Clint Black impressionist of some kind?* Walker was in the back seat and hadn't seen the sign, so we just tucked this into our astonished heads and decided to discuss it later.

"So Clint Black is appearing in Skokie," Ellen said later that night when Walker was asleep.

"Yes. I can't believe it," I said. "It's just too bad. He's such a hero to Walker."

"What do you mean 'just too bad'?" Ellen said.

"Well, Walker can't see him. We know he can't sit through concerts. He might not even sit for a whole song. Remember Vince Gill?" I was thinking of how, after we'd bought expensive tickets for a Vince Gill concert at Wrigley Field, Walker insisted on leaving the moment we sat down.

"Of course. I know. But I'm thinking maybe he could meet Clint Black, like before the concert."

Poor Ellen, I thought. *She's gone off the deep end. Next she'll want the Rolling Stones to come over to our house for coffee and bagels.*

"How would that happen?" I queried the fantasist.

"We ask," she said, and said it as if she knew what she was talking about.

The next day she ordered tickets for the two of us and sent off an email message to the North Shore Center about how she had an autistic son who adored Clint Black and wondered if he could meet the singer, just for a moment, before the concert. We waited two weeks and no reply. "Oh, well," I said. "It's a fine thing that you tried."

"Oh, I'm not done," she said.

Soon she telephoned them and did her Charming Ellen routine on the phone. As usual when she was talking, she sounded to me like she was chatting with an old dear friend. When she worked for a public relations firm long ago, one of her noted skills was, according to her boss, "giving good phone." Whenever a particularly tricky client had to be called, Ellen got the assignment. But this time, it didn't work. The guy at the other end was sympathetic but didn't think it could be done.

We brooded, hearts sinking.

But in another week the manager of the venue called us. Sure, he said, our son could meet Clint Black just before the concert. Come an hour before the concert and go to a door on the left in the lobby and we would be ushered in along with some other people.

→ ←

So we planned our Mission Impossible. Ellen and I would arrive with Walker at the appointed time. With iPhone watches synchronized by satellite, Dave and our tenant and friend, Allan, would arrive precisely one hour later to pick up Walker and take him home. Allan would drive; Dave would talk to Walker in the car. Ellen and I would then attend the concert. We thought this plan could work, though blueprints to the concert hall would have been reassuring. Where were entrances and exits in relation to the parking lots? How big was the lobby and how obvious was this "door on the left"?

Our biggest concern was this: Would Walker, at some point during the mission, just punt and demand to go home? Once he did that, there would be no stopping our six-foot-three son, and the whole clockwork plan would fall to pieces. As parents, we had evolved way past feeling embarrassed if he created a scene, but we did worry about our own broken hearts if it didn't work.

We prepared Walker as well as we could for the event and explained everything about the mission. He was happy and excited and understanding about the plan. Whenever we mentioned it, he smiled eagerly. We kept emphasizing how brief the meeting with Clint Black would be; we didn't want him to expect more than just a minute of rapture.

The day came. A happy hour-long ride in the car was followed by a happy entrance to the concert hall lobby. We felt as if we were just three normal adult fans walking normally into a normal busy lobby filled with other happy human normals. I never know how we really look. How quickly do people catch on to Walker's disability? When he's making a fuss or holding my hand, or when he's doing something odd like fluttering his hands fast down at his sides, I know people spot it right away. But sometimes when people look at him, I like to think that they just see a handsome young man and feel flattered when he smiles at them.

For some minutes we tried to fake good cheer and calm and looked around until we spotted "the door on the left" and some people near it with a certain facial glow, who looked like other Clint Black super fans about to be admitted to The Presence. Walker was cool and smiling, eyes sparkling with anticipation. Ellen and I were very, very nervous. Like the old Chicago Cub fans that we were, we aspired to hope for the best but we also steeled ourselves to be ready for the worst.

The friendly manager opened the door and motioned to all of us to enter. There were about 15 of us. I had a crazy thought:

Are all these people disabled? But nobody looked as if they had a problem like Walker did. *Maybe all of them have a connection of some kind to Clint Black?*

We walked down a long ramp and were ushered into a small basement area; the manager explained that Clint Black would come out in a few minutes and each of us would be able to take a photograph with him. Walker was by now grinning and doing a kind of all-body vibration. I was holding his right hand and whispering as calmly as I could to him. His left hand was shaking wildly in a modified air-guitar move. To everybody it was now obvious that a father was trying to keep his large son from rising to the ceiling with anticipation. I had a thought: *How often do performers have to deal with Spontaneous Fan Ascension?*

Ellen chatted a bit with the eager people around. One woman said that she and her husband had a special love of Clint Black because they had played a song of his at their wedding. We figured that most of the others had no more of a "connection" with Clint Black than a special request like hers and ours, and that this occasion was simply something he did to be nice to his fans. It was confirmation of a lesson my adviser once taught me in graduate school: "The people that get things in life, Bob, are the people who ask for them."

The manager spoke again after ten minutes had passed. "Clint will be here in five more minutes. You'll need to take turns and each person will have about a minute with Clint." "Five more minutes" was not good news. Walker was beginning to go "Ah, ah, ah!" loudly and started to pull me back up the ramp the way we had come. A woman came up to me and said, "Don't worry. I'm sure everybody here will let you go first." She was smiling and encouraging. I realized everybody around us was smiling and encouraging. It seemed that kindness was a requirement for initiation into the community of Clint Black superfans.

But Walker was tugging harder and starting to shout. Ellen said, her eyes getting tearful, "It's not gonna work. We might as well go." Another friendly superfan came up to her. "Would it help if I sang a Clint Black song to him? I'm a good singer. I know all his songs."

"Thanks," Ellen said. "But I don't think that would work right now."

The helpful idea was moot. I was now starting to wrestle with Walker. I pushed him away from the crowd toward a corner of the room that had a pop machine. I bought him a large Pepsi, but he wanted nothing to do with it. He started to yell, "Car!"

Ellen said, "It's no use. Let's go before there's more trouble."

After several minutes—an hour in Walker time—a representative for Clint emerged and said, "Five more minutes."

Ellen turned a despairing face to me.

Then a new identity took over my brain. I have no idea where this guy came from. It must be the same guy who takes over when test pilots calmly continue to play with the controls shortly before a crash. It was time for me to be Hero of the Day.

"He's not going anywhere," I said. "He's gonna see Clint Black if I have to sit on him. There's no way he's leaving this room. He's staying right here." I held him from behind with both arms. I talked to him firmly and quietly. He shouted and tugged at me, fighting to get away. He'd calm down for about ten seconds, but then rev right back up again. Eventually, it happened. A smiling, courtly man dressed all in black wearing a black cowboy hat emerged through a door. Walker immediately settled down. The crowd parted for Walker to take the first turn with the star.

As Ellen held the camera, Clint Black put his hand on Walker's back and said, "Hi, how you doin'?" He could see Walker was a special sort of fan and touched him delicately and calmly. Standing for the photo, Walker's feet were technically on the floor, but from the shoulders up he had clearly ascended. His idol was right there next to him, a hand on his back, just as real as Mom and Dad.

The rest of the mission went off without a hitch. Dave and Allan picked up the euphoric Walker on schedule, Ellen and I enjoyed the fabulous concert, and I felt like a leading-man dad straight out of Hollywood—maybe Liam Neeson in *Taken*?

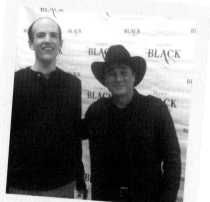

Walker and Clint Black

When he was seven or eight, Walker's favorite song was one that Clint Black recorded with Roy Rogers. Walker's speech teacher Maureen used to play it and dance with him at the end of every therapy session. It ended with the line, "If you hold on, partner / Good things are comin' to you / Hold on!"

I was beginning to realize these weren't just words of encouragement for the son; they were words the parents were starting to take to heart too.

CHAPTER 14

The Escape Artist

ON A SUNNY DAY in March, Walker and I stood clueless and nervous in the CHOICE program's central meeting room. The room was perfect in every way—so perfect that it seemed much too good for us. Brightly lit and newly furnished, it had the smell of just-painted walls in a freshly decorated room. The work table was behind us, reminding me of graduate classrooms in my long-ago days at Northwestern. We faced a huge Smart Board, the latest in classroom technology. I loved Smart Boards, a teaching tool just introduced at my school before I retired from teaching. I never learned to use them properly, but I had a lot of fun trying. It certainly must have dazzled Walker, who loved computers and especially his own iPad. But dazzling could also mean intimidating, and that was what was happening right now.

Walker had a remote in his hand and the friendly director of the program was inviting him to play a game. I can't remember exactly what the game was—maybe bowling? I can't remember because, like a car-crash victim who can't recall getting hit by the semi, I was traumatized. The friendly program director, a handsome, enthusiastic young man, had a tie on. A tie! No one at the agency had ever worn a tie, and I knew why. Every staff member had to be ready to wrestle gators at any moment. Dealing with clients like my son required a degree of physical prowess and rough-and-readiness. This man was dressed like a college teacher ready for a Wordsworth seminar.

Walker stood frozen, not knowing what to do with the remote. We'd always had difficulty getting Walker to participate in games. Even when he showed some initial skill, like kicking a soccer ball at a target, he'd eventually lose interest. "Losing interest" was what it always looked like, anyway, but we always wondered if it was fear: *If I do well at this, more and more will be expected of me until I can't do it at all. So I'll quit now.* This scenario of initial success followed by lack of interest was common with him. It had been true of ice skating, swimming, drawing, writing sentences, and especially speaking. When he started to talk at age one or so, his progress abruptly stopped as if talking was just an odd, random activity, like spelunking, that didn't interest him.

The director had invited Walker and me to come by for just an hour to get acquainted. But I knew, and I think Walker knew, that a lot more was at stake. The big question for Clearbrook and its CHOICE program was: Would this client fit? Would it work for him and us? It felt like a college interview that we were failing. *Oh my God*, I thought, *is this game something they regularly do here? Is this a sort of minimal test?* For Walker, it might as well be string theory. Up to now, all Clearbrook knew about Walker was what Ellen and I had told them (although we hoped that Mary and April from the Hope Institute had also been filling them in). This was their first look at the prospective client in the flesh. He wasn't showing the director any of the hidden intelligence and charm his parents had bragged about.

Walker was being cooperative and gentle, but he didn't look as if he had any actual abilities to work with.

When the hour was over, I felt as if we'd been tantalized with a glimpse of a better world we'd never be admitted to. Knowing what I knew about how terrible Walker's life at his last group home had been, how could he *not* bomb out of this program almost immediately? I knew, or thought that I knew, that he couldn't keep on an even keel here. Quiet seminar rooms are not for students who shout and bolt wildly into streets and scare the staff. But the director was still smiling when we left and still offered hope that maybe Walker could fit.

I didn't believe him.

→ ←

At home we worked with Walker like parents prepping Junior for the SAT with a view toward Ivy League applications. He'd always liked reading and writing, but his relationship with both had a troubled history. Unhappy with the public school special education programs we'd observed in the late 1980s and 1990s, we homeschooled Walker until age ten. We tried, hard, to give him a kind of "straight" schooling: buying and using books geared for first grade, second, third grade, and so on, and poring over good children's literature. But we also took his lead. He wanted—needed—to get outside and *move* every day. It was clearly a physical necessity with him. So I opted to teach my college classes at night (a wonderful aspect of my job: a flexible schedule) and hit the streets with him in the day, lecturing and pestering him with facts about the world around us. "Zoo–Train–Walk" was what remained of the most important "homeschooling" lesson of his childhood. But real, sit-down-with-a-book sessions had always been part of the routine.

These sessions were always problematic: sometimes delightful, sometimes excruciating. I could sit with him at his station at the dining-room table and lay out pennies for him to count, aspiring to addition and subtraction. One day he looked down at the pennies and said, "This is wonderful." It's not every day that a teacher gets that kind of feedback. On other days I could lay out some other groupings, maybe coins, maybe Hot Wheels cars—anything to count or lure him painlessly into mathematics—and he'd show interest before sweeping it all off the table and on to the floor with a swift movement of his arm. On these occasions, I'd have to dig deep into my small bank of strategies to control my temper, sometimes failing badly.

Once I hit upon a brilliant tutorial tactic. I set up a video camera on a tripod and taped our reading sessions. This went on for a whole summer. It had two benefits. The first was that he loved being photographed and taped; he was a star, he was important, he was being taken seriously. The lessons with a camera always lasted longer than without one. He was performing and showing off—dutifully doing his best. And he loved looking at the tapes later on TV. There he was, as real as Big Bird and all the characters that lived in that box. He once gave himself away and, nearly hugging the set, said, "I'm in the movie. I'm in the movie." In this he was merely following my lead, for I often abandoned the family and idled as a film extra whenever some production was in town. Later, we'd watch a movie together and I'd go, "See, I'm right there. No, not that guy, the other guy—the one behind the cop. Damn, can't you see?"

The other benefit was that I was on my best behavior. I never lost patience with the camera on. I was a perfect teacher, tireless in my attempts to introduce and reintroduce the material. When Walker would, at some random point, jump up and walk away from what we were doing, I'd cheerfully say, "OK, old man! That's about it for today, I guess." Watching my performances with him later in the replay, I often thought of the killer at the end of the Flannery O'Connor story "A Good Man is Hard to Find." He observes about his victim, "She would of been a good woman if it had been somebody there to shoot her every minute of her life." The same was true of me: put a camera in front of me and I'm a paragon of fatherhood.

The new sessions with writing and reading were just as revealing, euphoric, and maddening as the former ones had been. We'd work with the lists. He would say, as was his habit, "Write stuff down!" And we'd say, "No, man. *You* write stuff down." And we'd get out a laptop and start to work. He loved this, every time. "Where do we go first?" Ellen would say.

"Belmont Avenue," he'd reply.

"OK, write that."

Then he would write the two words unaided, or he would write the first three letters unaided and stop, or, more frequently, Ellen would slowly, tediously, announce each letter and he would hunt the letter down and strike the key. The hunting could be swift, as though automatic like that of a touch typist. Or it could be painfully slow, as though he'd never seen a keyboard before and was surprised at this newfangled invention—*Ya mean this here little thing'll write the dang letters for me?* His finger could hover over the letter he needed, say "t," and not come down. He'd look into Ellen's eyes, smiling. *Now where is that pesky letter?* he seemed to be saying. As with reading and writing and spelling and numbers all the years when he was growing up, the new writing sessions were all about *interaction*.

The relationship, the fun, the joke—these were what mattered, far more than the "lesson."

→ ←

So Walker's formal education was, and basically had always been, a bust. He would definitely not pass a test on reading, writing, and 'rithmetic. But where was the autism? Where was his penchant to be "off in a world of his own," his "object-, not person-orientation," his lack of empathy, his preference for abstraction, his lack of irony—all characteristics of the conventional wisdom about autistic people, none of which was visible in our tutorials? This was one of the big mysteries of his life. It was the main reason Ellen and I had been accused of being "in denial" about his condition when he was very young. In important ways, he just didn't act autistic.

This old enigma about him appeared rather dramatically late that winter. In our search for a new situation for him, his "packet of information" had to be updated: all his records from the agency plus his medical information plus his very label as "autistic." One day in March a young psychologist came over to the house to re-evaluate him. Walker loved this. A new person was coming over to talk to him? Yes! This might help him to get into a new home and voc program? Bring it on!

The psychologist, Jamal, was a friendly young man and Walker took to him immediately. He set up his testing materials on the dining-room table and, because Walker could not answer questions, he asked Ellen and me questions such as these:

Jamal: Does he make eye contact? (Conventional Wisdom: Not making eye contact is a very commonly held idea about autistics.)

Us: Yes, very much so. He can gaze into people's eyes. But sometimes, usually out of excitement, he has to avert his look.

Jamal: Does he prefer to be alone? (CW: "Alone" is basic to the very definition of autism.)

Us: Never. In the house, he's always in our faces, begging for attention. At his group home, they told us he liked to be alone in his room, but that was just to get away from violent housemates.

Jamal: Does he have special people that he likes? (CW: Autistics are object-oriented. They're much more comfortable with things—gadgets, toys, computers, puzzles—than with human society.)

Us: Very much so. His bonding with his speech teacher Maureen is the biggest one of his life. He calls our family physician, Dr. Weschler, his "best friend." The list could go on and on.

Jamal: Does he have a sense of humor? (CW: Jokes involve irony and autistic people are extremely literal. Think of the character Sheldon in *The Big Bang Theory*.)

Us: Yes, sometimes everything seems to be funny with him. A common joke: I sing silly words to songs he knows well. He doubles over with laughter.

Jamal: Is he afraid of crowds? (CW: Autistic people fear noise, need peace and quiet.)

Us: Yes and no. He walked eagerly and gladly with us over to the stupendously multitudinous Pride

Parade. After a short time, he was overwhelmed and had to leave. But we did too.

Jamal: Is he fearful of strangers? (CW: Autistic people do not like change. They like things to be orderly and predictable and therefore don't want a new cast of characters in their lives.)

Us: No, not at all. Look at how he received you today.

Jamal went on to give him a rudimentary IQ test. Some questions Walker answered straight, pointing correctly to the picture that didn't belong in the same set with the other pictures. Sometimes it was clear to us that Walker was kidding when he pointed to the obviously wrong picture, that he was teasing the new friend. All the time Walker was smiling, making very good eye contact, and was very relaxed.

When we eventually got his written report, Jamal had written, deadpan as it were, that Walker was *not* clearly autistic, that he had too many contraindications.

I waved the paper in my hands. "NOT AUTISTIC! He's cured! Cured at last! What's your problem, Mrs. Hughes?" I was shouting, "Your child is not autistic after all! Medical and psychological science were just joking! Ha ha!"

Of course, we knew Walker had autism and that the "conventional wisdom"—medical science as filtered through network news and newspapers and blogs—was not the current best understanding of the condition. But it was often the way it played out in the real world. We knew that the grasp of autism by group-home staff and teachers and even some doctors (and psychologists) was actually well *below* the conventional wisdom.

The key characteristics of Walker's condition are a crippling inability to communicate, an obsession with schedules and routine, anxiety about the unknown immediate future, a tendency to be overwhelmed with emotion, and an inability to focus related to apparent huge distraction in his head. (This last one is vague, but it's the best I can do. It hits me very often throughout my days with him.) His type of autism is a real monster. It's not, as some might have it, a badge of membership in a proud community. It's the tragedy of his life.

→ ←

Would Clearbrook accept him? The prospect that he might get in seemed remote to us. The voc program, CHOICE, seemed geared for higher-functioning clients. The group home in the sleepy suburb we'd visited seemed too good to be true: quiet, attractive, and geared for a steadier, more tranquil sort of person, not our challenging son. But, amazingly, Clearbrook continued to show interest, and a group of four people from its administrative staff were scheduled to drop by for a home visit.

Of course, this meant Family Panic was the order of the day. If Walker could hold it together for this visit the way he had for April and Mary, all might be well. Nothing was a sure thing, of course, but if this visit was successful, we'd move on to a next step. However, if he carried on the way the agency had insisted he did—that he was now a "changed" person who required stiff discipline and staff trained in martial arts—well, *aloha* on a steel guitar to the Hugheses. At least this was the anxious way we framed the meeting to ourselves, and this panicky sense of the meeting's importance was what we tried to hide from Walker but probably communicated to him anyway.

On the day of the meeting, we set the living-room area up as usual. Square pie was ready in the refrigerator. Cheese pizza was in the oven. The usual puzzles were stacked nearby. Walker was nicely dressed and patient. The doorbell rang and in walked four smiling people, two men and two women.

This was when Walker miraculously put on a charm offensive like we'd never seen before. He walked over to them and said "Hi," then sat down on the couch next to one of the women, Emily. He proceeded to give her the love-at-first-sight treatment, gazing into her eyes and grinning merrily. After some time, he went over to the table and had his square pie and pizza, then decided to work the male part of his audience. He picked up the TV remote and said to one of the men, Dave, "Basketball?" It was March Madness and Walker knew daytime games were on television. He had no real interest in basketball. He never suggested to us that he wanted to watch it, and turned off the TV when it was on. But for them it was *Hey, us guys, we watch basketball, right?* He was playing the smooth host, the ready-for-prime-time adult young man. The performance took our breath away.

And his new persona continued to amaze. At the CHOICE program, they invited him to come on his first day for just two hours. After all, if he behaved the way he had at the agency, he could be very disruptive. Ellen and I dropped him off at the site in Evanston and nervously sat across from each other at an Evanston Starbucks, drinking coffee and steeling ourselves for disaster. But it didn't come. When we picked him up, they reported that he was cooperative, quiet, and very cheerful. We drove back home with him to Wrigleyville via an ice-cream stop at the Happiest Place on Earth, the Lincolnwood Town Center Mall. We couldn't praise him enough. For a week, he went to the program for just two hours a day. Then he went for three hours. When he finally graduated to all day, including lunch, we began to know hope.

The basic principle of the program was that students could actually choose among a variety of activities that were available from day to day. Walker's favorite was "Meals on Wheels" (which he always referred to as "Wheels on Wheels"). He rode in a van that delivered food to shut-ins. The boxes with meals were closed and not easily opened—a convenient fact, for Walker was a food thief extraordinaire—and he rode in the truck with an aide. This combined many favorite things for him: physical movement, meeting new people, feeling useful, getting outdoors.

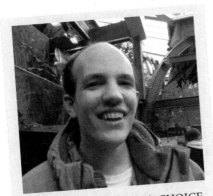

Walker on a field trip with CHOICE

At first, Walker's main activity was the one developed in the psych ward and at home: watching music videos on his iPad. The staff indulged him here. He was able to sit with the others and navigate his country hits at will. But after some months passed by, he no longer wanted anything to do with the iPad but preferred to play games and get out with others on field trips.

One "chosen" activity was especially marvelous for him: speech therapy with his oldest friend, Maureen Sweeney. Maureen had been a kind of family savior to us when Walker was very young. We had looked hard for professional help for him outside the Chicago Public School special ed system and finding her gave all of us hope for Walker. She became what he needed all along: a trusted friend and therapist who made him feel good about himself. Maureen had tried often to see Walker at his group home and volunteered to give free speech therapy sessions to clients at the CILA. But in spite of her wonderful reputation in the autism community, she was always rebuffed by the agency. Staff there had a suspicion—a well-founded one in retrospect—that outside people would not be impressed by the way they handled their clients. CHOICE, however, welcomed her and encouraged Walker to see her for therapy sessions. So he "chose" to go to Maureen's office on Thursdays when others were scheduled to go to a farm.

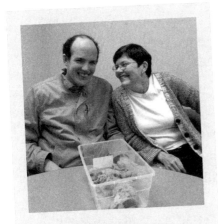

Walker and Maureen

Maureen sent us a photo from their first meeting. Walker was vibrating so much with happy excitement that he couldn't take his jacket off at first.

The CHOICE program was clearly doing something very right. We became accustomed to a new, wide, calm smile on his face each day when we picked him up.

↝ ↜

The last step would be his entry to the group home, which wouldn't be ready for him until October 1st. We wondered all through the summer and into the fall: Would he accept the idea of living there? Had he gotten too used to living with his parents again? Shouldn't he be suspicious of the group home lifestyle concept?

The house was a little over an hour away from our place in Chicago. So it became a frequent drive-by destination on our car trips with him. We'd drive up to the house, a ranch-style place on a corner with huge trees all around. We would stop and talk about how he was going to move in there on October 1st. He'd have a room of his own and two other housemates. He would ride in a van from the house to the CHOICE program each day. He loved to ride and would love the hour's drive back and forth to Evanston from the house.

One day we stopped by his old CILA home to get one more bag of his stuff. We had cleared out all his things weeks before, but they had found some more of his clothes among others in the confusing mix of the residents' laundry. I parked the car and Ellen dashed in the front door to get his things. Walker, who a couple of years ago would have raced happily into the house, didn't even attempt to get out of the car. When Ellen returned, he said, "House!"

"You mean your new house? The one you'll move into in October?" Ellen said.

"House!" he shouted again. He wanted to be reassured: *This place where Mom just went is history, right?*

"Sure," I said. "Let's go to the house."

→ ←

When the end of September came, we couldn't suppress our concern. We knew Walker was doing very well. He had gained weight and looked the picture of health. His smile had returned but it had an extra *edge* to it—a more knowing, adult look—

and he smiled this way virtually all of the time. One day when we picked him up at CHOICE, a staff member told us, "He's the happiest person I've ever known." His most notable quality all of his life had been his joy. It was his great blessing—a wonderful plus in life for him, and an inspiration to his parents. Now others could see it again and wondered at it too.

He was back. But one question remained: How would he do at his new home? After months of living at home with us, the big day, October 1st, arrived. The plan was for us to take him to CHOICE in the morning. Then at the end of the day a van would take him to his new group home. We talked to him endlessly about what would happen and he seemed to understand. That morning when we came down the stairs to get breakfast, he was already up, still in his pajamas, but with one shoe on and his lunchbox in his hand.

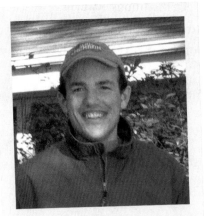

Walker in front of his new group house

He was ready and he was eager.

He took to his new house as the most natural thing in the world. When we picked him up on Saturday and Sunday mornings, he was eager to go home and run around the city. When he returned each Saturday and Sunday evening, he was just as eager to get back to his house, his bedroom. He wanted this and, we think, had been dreaming of this all along.

→ ←

In the novel *Catch-22*, there is a character called Orr who seems like a catastrophically bad World War II bomber pilot. In mission after mission, he crashes his plane but miraculously survives. At the end of the book, however, it turns out that he's the cleverest pilot of them all. All his crashes were intentional test runs preparatory to making a grand escape from the hell that was the war. In his last crash, he escapes into the sea on a life raft and rows his way to Sweden, a neutral country where he was safe.

Sometimes Walker's odyssey seems like Orr's to me. He couldn't tell anyone what he wanted or needed or was feeling. So he employed everything he could—his body, his voice, his hands, his expressions—to mime and push and pull his way out of a bad situation and into a better one. He was clearly the "worst" client at his old house. But so much of what happened could be interpreted as calculation on his part. As a client at the agency, he seemed as if he'd bottomed out, and his behavior in the CILA seemed intolerable (but intentionally so?). So they sent him to the psych ward (exactly the result he wanted). When he got back to the CILA, he went into his closet and refused to move (intentional intolerable behavior again). So his parents took him home (the result he wanted: he's happy now). April and Mary come to the house (yes!—friends who can help him move to a better place). April and Mary leave (he's still home—good; but he's not in a new place yet—bad, his behavior is mixed). His parents look for a new group home and voc program for him (*finally, you're getting the idea, people!*). He's extra charming to every visitor but only middling charming with his parents (easy to interpret now). He finally gets his way: new voc and a new house = happiness (*thanks, everybody*).

I can imagine him saying:

Well, that's an exaggeration, Dad. When I was at the CILA, I was just panicked. I was out of my mind with hopelessness. I knew I could get hurt any time. I knew the staff didn't like me. Nobody was friendly. My friends had all turned on me. I didn't even want to eat. I wasn't planning anything. But you're partly right. I did intentionally put on my best behavior for the visitors. I knew they were my ticket out. So I poured it on. It was a little bit of an act, I guess, but the panic at the CILA was no act. And I like new people. I like anybody who's nice. I would have talked to them a lot if I could. I do know when it's important to be friendly and I thought about that when the visitors came. So I steered you a little.

But there was no plan.

His reception of the Clearbrook visitors, his intentional pouring on of the charm and honest delight in meeting people who wished him well—all of it was a revelation to Ellen and me. We had always been his biggest fans, his cheerleaders, always finding positives in his character where many others saw merely negatives.

But even we had underestimated him. This young man, wild with anxiety, nevertheless could think and act more prudently than his loving boosters knew. He was more than friendly and smart and loving. He was resilient.

CHAPTER 15

Afterword

July 2015

WE ARE LUCKY PEOPLE, we Hugheses.

I say this despite the superstitious feeling that the words invite doom on our heads. I think of Bart Simpson saying to his father, "This is the worst day of my life," and Homer, reliably horrible, replying, "The worst day of your life *so far*." Maybe a qualification is needed. Considering the world that families with autism face—so far anyway—we are very, very lucky.

A few of our blessings:

Clearbrook appeared and accepted Walker just when we needed it. In the state of Illinois, this is something of a miracle. April and Mary and the Hope Institute were of great help in alerting the Illinois Division of Developmental Disabilities to the dire situation Walker was in. In addition, the director of Clearbrook thought that Walker would be a good fit for the new CHOICE program he was starting; at the same time, an opening in a group home was appearing that seemed to be a match for Walker's temperament.

Another blessing was the good fortune that Ellen and I happened to look at Walker's problems the same way. In fact, the challenge has been something that keeps us together (so far!). Before marriage, we asked the same vitally important questions that other couples do: "Do we like the same movies? The same music? Are we in love? OK, let's go!" We didn't ask of the spousal candidate: "In the event of a disabled child, what course would you wish to take?" That Ellen and I agreed when push came to shove was sheer, blind luck. We were saved from the stark fact that many couples split over differences they have in regard to a disabled child.

A huge blessing was my job. I worked at a secure college teaching post for 37 years and was required to be at the school only about six hours a day, Fridays off. I had a flexible schedule and thus the opportunity to get to know my sons in ways fathers who work 12-hour days never experience. Ellen quit her public relations job and early on worked at freelance grant writing. This enabled her to be at home all the time, bearing the main brunt (and the main joy) of being with the boys. But this assured income was lucky. Unemployment hits a big portion of the workforce and hurts families unpredictably.

The biggest blessing has been Walker's happy nature. His default position is a smile. This did not have to be. People with autism are like everyone else, with the full spectrum of personality. They can be happy or depressed, relaxed or irritable, friendly or introverted, funny or serious. Walker's good nature can smooth over rough situations, and the rough situations have come in swarms over the years.

Yet with all our luck, all our education, child-orientedness, and steady middle-middle-class income, Walker almost fell through the cracks.

Why? There were many factors at work, but a very big one was money. In the U.S. there is, more or less, decent financial support for special education students up through age 21. The "No Child Left Behind" idea garners widespread support. After all, who's not for helping kids? But when a child becomes an adult, that magical support crumbles. In Illinois, it crumbles shamefully.

As I write, Illinois is ranked 48th in the U.S. in its aid to disabled people, out of the 50 states plus the District of Columbia. Shockingly, this number is too good to many in the state who fight hard politically to push that number higher. Every decent group home or agency—each with a long waiting list of families in need of services—is continually threatened by more and more cuts in funding. The result is that there are many disabled adults living at home with aging parents who live in severe anxiety about what will happen to their child.

Adults with disabilities just don't generate the interest that children do. Children are cute. And some children, according to a good number of memoirs, are "cured" in one dramatic way or another. Such happy story arcs are very attractive and exciting. But adults with low-functioning autism plummet very far below our media radar. Most of them, like Walker, can't perform viral YouTube-type stunts: play a Beethoven sonata, shoot winning baskets in a basketball game, or sing "The Star-Spangled Banner." Most of them can't say or do things that quickly connect with others and establish that elusive thing we think of as "worth." And when this connection isn't there, people—that is, taxpayers—don't like to think about this needy population growing older and less cute. Thus, society can and does fail the critical test of providing financial help to its most needy citizens.

In this book, I've focused much of the blame for Walker's mistreatment on certain people at his agency. But behind the staff's failures was the pressure of financial constraint. Walker's first years at the CILA and the voc program were good, even better than the norm, because the staff he came in contact with happened to be smart, dedicated, loving people. But the agency was small and had trouble paying the people who worked there. It didn't help that the state of Illinois was very bad at providing funds for any agencies for the disabled in any sort of timely fashion. So when good staff moved on to other work or careers, there was no guarantee that equally good people would replace them. Underpaid, low-status work such as this only attracts good people when there is thoughtful education for job candidates and a canny screening process. And such a process costs money. Walker's world fell apart because of the natural entropy of a small, financially strapped organization. Clearbrook by contrast is a large, well-funded, and, for the adult disabilities world, "prosperous" organization. Its fine ethos doesn't depend on the luck of good hires here and there: professional education and screening guarantee a strong staff.

I've written this book because nobody would pay attention to me if I stood with a megaphone at the corner of State and Randolph Streets in Chicago, shouting, "My son and others like him are worthwhile people! Get to know them! Make friends with them! Your life will be enriched! And pass laws that will help them lead satisfying lives!" Or, come to think of it, maybe people would pay attention in ways that would surprise me. It could be worth a try, actually.

→ ←

It's a warm summer Saturday and Walker and I are Zoo–Train–Walking again, this time with gratifyingly few index-card lists.

We've seen our friends, the cashiers at Starbucks and Walgreens, and gorged on croissants and ice-cream cones (I'm joining him today on every treat—I mean, why not?), and we've passed a huge number of pink-shirted cancer walkers along the path to the Lincoln Park Lagoon. Ahead lies the boardwalk, a treat on our long treks. Over a few years and many many walks, we watched them build this marvelous walkway. First they drained the lagoon. Then they imbedded large posts all over the place. We constantly wondered from week to week, and sometimes from day to day, *What the heck are they doing here?*

The answer was this long, zig-zaggy plank sidewalk over carefully planned and lovely wetland vegetation. Everywhere there are birds, sometimes rather exotic ones, but normally the four I write down on an index card every time we approach. This time is no exception: "Ducks–geese–seagulls–red-winged blackbirds."

Holding my hand, Walker tugs me along and I have some difficulty keeping up. He glances at his current index card. Then he looks out at the water. Sure enough, there they all are, or at least three of them. The seagulls are swooping and talking in their goofy and alarming way. The geese are honking and flying in squadrons and landing on the water in the distance. Small duck nuclear families are swimming near the boardwalk itself, looking for treats from likely human marks. Today there are also a large number of crows putting up a big squawk. Walker turns and looks at me and smiles as if we share an in-joke about these guys. His look says something more to me: *I love getting out here with you. Thanks, Dad.* Then he gazes out at the water again, forward at the tall water grasses ahead of us, and upward at the sky, grinning.

When I was in college long ago, I first read a poem by e.e. cummings that, as time went by and living furnished the words with more and more meaning, I learned to cherish. The first verse goes:

> I thank You God for most this amazing day:
> for the leaping greenly spirits of trees
> and a blue true dream of sky...

In Walker's eyes, trees do leap greenly, the sky really is a blue true dream, and even his dad, some of the time anyway, is a most amazing fellow. His insight is a gift that he gives quite casually to me and other people in his life. He manages to do this despite great obstacles: the continuous noise in his head, the outsize fears nobody else understands, the frustration of rarely finding the words for his thoughts.

This is it, I often think. This is the kind of courage life requires, and this is the kind of love that pulls us through.

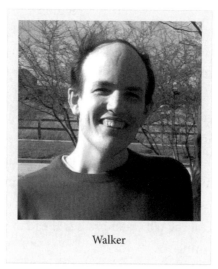

Walker